THE TOWN SLOWLY EMPTIES

ON LIFE AND CULTURE DURING LOCKDOWN

MANASH FIRAQ BHATTACHARJEE

HEADPRESS

A HEADPRESS BOOK
First published by Headpress, Oxford, UK, in 2020
headoffice@headpress.com

THE TOWN SLOWLY EMPTIES
On Life And Culture During Lockdown

Text copyright © MANASH FIRAQ BHATTACHARJEE
Foreword © SASHA DUGDALE
This volume copyright © HEADPRESS 2020
Cover photo copyright © ABDULLAH SAGHIR AHMAD : Instagram @the.final.shot
Cover design MARK CRITCHELL : mark.critchell@googlemail.com : graphixengine.co.uk
Book layout & design GANYMEDE FOLEY
Proofing : JENNIFER WALLIS

10 9 8 7 6 5 4 3 2 1

The moral rights of the author have been asserted.

The views expressed in this publication do not necessarily reflect the views of the publisher.

All Rights Reserved. No part of this book may be reproduced, stored in a retrieval system, or transmitted, in any form or by any means, electronic, mechanical, photocopying, recording or otherwise, without prior permission in writing from the publisher.

A CIP catalogue record for this book is available from the British Library

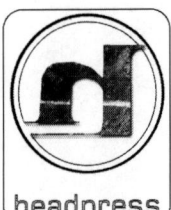

ISBN   978-1-909394-75-9 (paperback)
ISBN   978-1-909394-76-6 (ebook)
NO-ISBN (hardback)

HEADPRESS. POP AND UNPOP CULTURE.

Exclusive NO-ISBN special edition hardbacks and other items of interest are available at HEADPRESS.COM

Praise for the book

"In this book of quiet meditations, Manash Firaq Bhattacharjee shows the unique value of sensible, informed and honest thought in a world torn apart by religion and politics in the grip of a serious pandemic. Ordinary acts — what you cook for breakfast, advice on how to obtain wine, friendship and love, poetry, thinking about flowers and grass — such things enter a sequence alongside the plight of destitute workers, the meaning of masks… The greatest contribution is the author's sheer calm of mind in a world driven mad by anxiety."

~ Peter Riley, Editor of *The Fortnightly Review*

"What does a poet and an intellectual do when 'the world had turned into a zoo' and 'no visitors were allowed in'? Manash Firaq Bhatatcharjee follows numerous fine examples from world literature. They all share an ethical necessity to remain awakened through language, to write and to chronicle in times of severe grief and tragedy. In his diary from the first three weeks of the surge of Covid-19 in India, Manash interweaves captivating observations, piercing personal memories and essayistic reflections with a double goal: to bear witness and to remain a human being."

~ Aleš Steger, Author of *Above the Sky Beneath the Earth*

"Lyrical and evocative, this is a pandemic journal with a difference. Deftly capturing the passing of slow lockdown time in an India otherwise devoted to speed and violence, it demands that we partake in the restorative powers of love, literature, and well-cooked fish."

~ Siddhartha Deb, Author of *The Beautiful and the Damned: Life in the New India*

"Manash Firaq Bhattacharjee negotiates the Covidocene, navigating through an everyday experience rendered radically unrecognisable by pandemic. What sustains the narrator-protagonist of this beautiful and compelling memoir of our very own plague year is his passionate, full-bodied immersion in culture. Even as he engages with the quotidian acts of survival around him, he endows them with the sumptuous, unpredictable beauty and sublimity of the poetry and fiction he has read, the films he has seen, the food he has known as folk memory, recipe and dish. The besieged imagination, which, as Manash reminds us, is both an aesthetic and a political force, refuses to renounce its resilient, intransigent mobility."

~ Ranjit Hoskote, Author of *The Atlas of Beliefs*

"This is a remarkable work in many ways — whether in terms of the sheer quality of the writing or the way in which the writer combines an account of the material reality of lockdown with history, literature and philosophy. The cultural criticism is breathtaking in its range."

~ Keshava Guha, Author of *Accidental Magic*

'Toward two o'clock the town slowly empties, it is the time when silence, sunlight, dust, and plague have the streets to themselves.'

Albert Camus, *The Plague*

To the eucalyptus tree beside my terrace
for its rustle of leaves, birds and ancient company

Contents

FOREWORD by Sasha Dugdale	1
PREFACE Nature Is Elsewhere	3
NEWSPAPERS, PLAGUES, FISH & IMMORTALITY	
Monday, March 23	13
OF CHILDREN & MOTHERS IN A TIME OF FORGETTING	
Tuesday, March 24	27
TREES, FORESTS & THE FOX'S WEDDING	
Wednesday, March 25	33
WE FEAR BRAVELY	
Thursday, March 26	40
THE DISEASE ARRIVED VIA AEROPLANES	
Friday, March 27	48
MRS. DALLOWAY'S FLOWERS & THE GRASS AT PURANA QILA	
Saturday, March 28	52
COPPER COINS & ABSTRACT SHIT	
Sunday, March 29	64
GRATITUDE IS THE HEAVIEST DEBT	
Monday, March 30	72
OF MASKS, MONTAIGNE, ALCOHOL & FRIENDSHIPS	
Tuesday, March 31	76
THE CRUELLEST MONTH & FOOD AS APHRODISIAC	
Wednesday, April 1	85
LIGHT THE CANDLES	
Thursday, April 2	93
DEATH, FAMINE & MORALITY IN SATYAJIT RAY'S FILMS	
Friday, April 3	99

"Trust Begets Trust"
   Saturday, April 4 — 104

Chernobyl, Bhopal & the Gospel of Reason
   Sunday, April 5 — 110

Memory, History & the Tunnel of Schoolmates
   Monday, April 6 — 119

Of Moustaches, Forgotten Clothes & Sadness
   Tuesday, April 7 — 126

The Absence of Absence
   Wednesday, April 8 — 136

Treatise for the Wanderer & the Colour of Waiting
   Thursday, April 9 — 143

On Love: Razia Begum, Shakespeare, Kiarostami
   Friday, April 10 — 146

Rome on the Balcony
   Saturday, April 11 — 152

Dilshad Mohammad, Yannis Ritsos, Jafar Panahi
   Sunday, April 12 — 156

Of Sleep, Dreams & Insomnia
   Monday, April 13 — 162

To Cross or Not Cross the Line
   Tuesday, April 14 — 171

Select bibliography & filmography — 179
Notes — 183
Index — 196
About the author — 200

Foreword

by Sasha Dugdale

THE TOWN SLOWLY EMPTIES, MANASH FIRAQ'S LYRICAL DIARY OF lockdown in India, opens like a flower, drawing the reader in. I find myself reading the short essay-chronicles obsessively, entranced by the combination of poetry, beauty, poverty and pandemic.

Despite Manash's learnedness and wealth of references, the text retains a raw and authentic tone, describing an experience from the inside, unmediated by time and memory. And yet the interweaving of poetry, politics and meditation (and wonderful food), suggest that it's a text which has long been on the author's mind — the product of many years of thought-connection, but given play and shape by the conditions of lockdown and an unprecedented freedom to follow the meandering rhythms of the mind, and to project all this light and colour out into a drab and deserted world.

Manash's personal history and the history of a nation, a people and a civilisation are aligned in each chapter, as if this moment when everything is silent and empty and open has permitted this seeping through of the past. The journal-style allows a degree of freedom to move above and tackle what concerns the writer on any given day, what he might see from his window, or a conversation he has had with a friend. Concerns and themes run through the text, growing in potency and complexity and handed on from day to day, like motifs, to resound ever more fully.

I admire Manash's ability to discuss political and philosophical issues, whilst preserving a lightness of touch and poetic ease: to combine intense seriousness and compassion, to analyse a poem in depth and respond to it, and then immediately indulge in laughter and sensuousness; the wonderful comparison of friendship and spices he produces as an aside — which I will forever use as a guide to both friends and cooking spices; the relatives and street characters who people his pages; nothing is off bounds for the roving authorial eye. The observations are delightful and provocative and sad and wistful. Nor does he eschew the hard truths of the pandemic, its politics and the ways it hits the poor. Some of his most heartfelt passages are condemnations of politics and nationalism and deeply compassionate towards the disenfranchised and hopeless.

Most of all, I feel at home in the internationalism of the book. The reach of Manash's allusions and his cultural touchstones make the book feel like a point in a network of cultures, a republic of letters and films and politics. It was something I could grasp and share from this distant place, as much as the experience of disease and lockdown. When Manash takes an Eastern European poet and reads his poem as it speaks to him and his situation in India, in a pandemic which touches us all, I was moved to return to the poems I love and consider them again — as torches to light us through this dark period in our collective history.

Preface:
Nature Is Elsewhere

Today is 23 June. It has been one long, endless day since 23 March, when the nationwide lockdown began in India. Life has increasingly grown passive. We don't seem to use the days. Days use us. Our activities have been reduced to circling inside our homes. Life has been reduced to a few rooms. There is suddenly an anxious gulf between inside and outside, home and the world. The world is thrust into a new time, one that will usher in visible and invisible changes, and significantly alter our idea of life.

The atmosphere in the city of Delhi, free from the pollution of daily traffic, has cleared. Everyone is struck by the fresh blueness of the sky and the clarity of the stars at night. Like us, the trees and birds look refreshed from breathing a cleaner air. Prior to this, with total disregard for life and environment, human indulgence pumped hazardous elements into nature. The lockdown has helped the fog of pollution to lift. It needed human beings to be forced out of the streets like unruly children, for the atmosphere to begin cleaning up the mess.

The accident that caused the outbreak of the coronavirus pandemic has released a set of logical consequences: death, health emergency, forced isolation, social distancing and paranoia. In India, the outbreak also caused two unanticipated consequences: a decrease in pollution levels particularly in cities, and the huge reverse migration of daily wage labourers from cities to their homes in small towns.

The coronavirus pandemic reaffirmed the view of those who believe that history is never linear and unfolds in unpredictable ways.

T.S. Eliot writes in *Gerontion*, 'Think / Neither fear nor courage saves us.'[1] Eliot says this in the context of history and how it deceives us with 'cunning passages'.[2] It is a necessary warning. The key word here is 'think' — an invitation to reflect.

Under lockdown, the radically new experience of life provokes us not to succumb to our usual, human propensities. This warning is useless for the migrant labourers whose daily earnings have suddenly disappeared as they face a situation of imminent hunger. They are forced to take a risk whose consequences they are not always capable of overcoming. Many have died of hunger or met with inexplicably cruel accidents on their way home. The health workers also risked their lives to attend to Covid-19 patients and many have been infected and died.

But for the rest of us who are a little guilty of the luxury — however stifling — of home and yet not saved from restless anxieties, reflection is an ethical necessity.

||

As COVID-19 CAUGHT the world unawares, human interaction was suddenly insecure and the future uncertain. In such moments, one takes a flight to the past. Childhood suddenly becomes visible. Not the nostalgia but the enigma of childhood. The road to adulthood is paved with strange flowers. These are flowers one cannot name.

The lockdown also prompted renewed interaction with nature. The sudden disruption of life's mechanised routine and the conventional, daily ties with the world, led people to look elsewhere. There they found nature.

Those who could afford fancy mobile phones took pictures of birds and trees with newfound excitement and posted these on Instagram and other social media. It was a departure from the habit of oblivion that is imbued in modern, fast-paced life.

This accidental love of and return to nature was one undertaken under duress. It may remain transitory. Transitory passion is the essence of modern existence. People have been treating the environment like a commode: both, by a physical flushing out of the trees around them and flushing them out of memory.

In Abbas Kiarostami's film *Taste of the Cherry* (1997), we see tractors and dump trucks at various excavation sites, as the distressed protagonist, Homayoun Ershadi, drives through Tehran. The sites rupture the greenness with the colour of excavated rocks and stones. The sudden chirping of birds against the constant noise of automation reminds one of the erosion of nature.

There is a poem by Vinod Kumar Shukla, 'Sheher Se Sochta Hun' (I Think from the City) whose first lines read:

I think from the city,
is the forest being cut even from my imagination?
If the forest can't be in the forest,
where will it be?
It will be in the trees, in the corner of city streets.[3]

It may remind readers of the Aarey forest controversy in Mumbai, where 3,000 trees are to be felled and relocated to make space for building a car shed for the Metro. The matter is currently in the courts, though around 2,000 trees have already been cut. The growing population of cities needs more space for travel. Trees are expendable.

|||

CHARLES BAUDELAIRE HERALDED the modern era in his famous essay of 1863, 'The Painter of Modern Life.' He called modernity an 'indefinable something' and its exemplary figure, someone who is forever 'quickening his pace... forever in search'.[4] This figure is different from Baudelaire's other, celebrated figure of the *flâneur*, the spectator of modern life from the sidelines.

The modern self, instead, is looking for a quality it cannot name. Modernity is a name for the unnameable. It is, Baudelaire says, 'the transient, the fleeting'.[5] Everyone is rushing towards what is disappearing, rushing towards their own disappearance.

This rushing is not just individual. It is collective. It has a structural dimension.

The idea of 'progress' holds sway. Life is at the mercy of a mad, accumulative project. We are being forced to rediscover human leisure today. Leisure is often marked by a paradoxical mode of experience. You are hooked and distracted, as you fleetingly pass through images that appear on your smartphone or on billboards in the plaza. The elsewhere is *here*, digitally fed into your imagination.

The idea of human progress was defined in quantifiable terms. This was due to the triple effect of capitalism, science and technology, each contributing to a rational meaning of human life. The idea of life mirrored the logic of production: the maximization of happiness (an idiotic idea propounded by Jeremy Bentham[6]) corresponded to the maximization of goods. We were to measure our values, in true utilitarian manner, against numbers. The index of happiness, associated with wealth, goods and property, became a value.

Baudelaire had summed up this all-encompassing utilitarian obsession with precision: 'All is Number. Number is in all. Number is in the individual. Ecstasy is a Number.'[7]

The worldwide death toll due to Covid-19 appears in a list that is constantly updated. *Death has become a table of growing numbers.* People are dying in numbers.

IV

ISOLATION DURING THIS pandemic has united people like never before. We live in a world alienated from itself, by its routine of work and its dictated pleasures, distancing from others simply because the timetable that pays our bills insists on buying our time. We pretend to live in our own time, but we live in a time whose hours are fixed by others.

Albert Camus writes in *The Plague*, 'The common lot of married couples. You get married, you go on loving a bit longer, you work. And you work so hard that it makes you forget to love.'[8]

Faiz Ahmed Faiz, in his poem 'kuchh ishq kiya kuchh kaam kiya' wrote something similar:

hum jeete-ji masroof rahe
kuchh ishq kiya kuchh kaam kiya
kaam ishq ke aade aata raha
aur ishq se kaam ulajhta raha
phir aakhir tung aakar hum ne
dono ko adhoora chhod diya

I was busy as long as I lived.
I loved a bit, worked a bit.
Work came in the way of love.
And love created obstacles in work.
Finally, in exasperation,
I left both unfinished.[9]

Our mechanised work culture[10] leaves people little time to pursue the calling of their heart. Even Faiz, being a poet, admitted he could not escape the clutches of 'productivity'.

We are subjected to a binary of existence that is real and absurd at the same time. The world of social media, often masquerading as one of remote solidarities, has deepened the chasm between people without us realising it.

In such a world, the phrase 'social distancing' cannot be more alien (or alienating). But the reason behind social distancing in this instance was to avoid a pandemic. It created the expected ripples of anxiety and fear. Paranoia comes easily to a world that feeds on it daily. Our social and personal relations are estranged in multiple ways.

We are not just estranged from the world, but from ourselves.

If we are bound to remain, to live and die as conflicted creatures of nature, it is even more necessary to understand how to live bearably within these conflicts. These and other contradictions are perfect matters to reflect upon in the days that open before me like empty roads. I took upon this unending day of enforced isolation as a moment to look back upon life and the world. Even if we landed here by a freak accident, it was caused by us. Thinking is an act of responsibility, where we have less excuses to falter. We err in our acts all the time. We haven't learnt to act the way we think. To again refer to Eliot, this time from *The Hollow Men*: 'Between the idea / And the reality/ ... Falls the shadow.'[11]

Reason tends to justify what we do. It is inherently self-driven. Its prime motivations are selfish. Scientific reasoning weighs on trial and error. What is good for studying objects may not be good for us. Science is a kind of technology, but human beings aren't science. We are a technology more complex and vulnerable than science. Our technology is closer to the technology of nature, and as enigmatic.

Gandhi famously spoke out against modern machinery in his book, *Hind Swaraj*, written in 1909 in the form of a Socratic dialogue, where an editor responds to questions from a reader. But Gandhi's position on the subject is more nuanced than what is generally understood to be a complete rejection of modern technology. Replying to a question about his aversion to machinery, Gandhi said, "I know that even this body is a most delicate piece of machinery [?] The spinning wheel is a machine; a little toothpick is a machine. What I object to is the craze for machinery, not machinery as such."[12] He added, "The machine should not be allowed to cripple the limbs of man."[13] Gandhi understands the human body as a kind of technology. He draws a distinction between the body's fragile technology and technology as a tool of mechanical power over the human body. He makes it clear that he is only averse to the fetish of machinery, not machinery "as such". Gandhi is arguing against a cult of technology, made possible by science.

We need to move away from reason and think from our heart. There are more mysterious and ethical ways of understanding ourselves and the world. The character Hossein in Abbas Kiarostami's film, *Through the Olive Trees* (1994), spoke about his heartbreak. The mother of Tahereh, the girl he pined for, turned down his marriage proposal. The same night an earthquake ravaged Koker, a farming village in northern Iran, and took the lives of Tahereh's parents. Hossein compared the earthquake to "the sighing of my heart". By drawing a seismic connection between the tremor of the land and his heart, Hossein draws upon our deeper relationship with land and nature, something not ethnic or territorial, but human. It illuminates our poetic understanding of life, more beautifully than reason.

V

THE MYSTERIOUS FEARS and isolation of a pandemic can trigger memory. You are more intensely drawn to the life you lived, in the face of uncertainty and danger. It is no wonder then that I was pulled back in time to recapitulate my ties with childhood, places visited in another era, to half-forgotten streets and people, like images from an old film.

Writing too is an activity that is aided by constraints. I had nowhere to go, no one to ask for a meeting, and nothing much to do. Forced to grapple with an extended state of isolation, the act of writing gained an intensity I had not encountered before. The body is forced into confinement, but the mind is free to soar.

VI

THE DAYS PRECEDING the lockdown have a strange, blurry quality. They were the last days of relative sanity, and what we inaccurately call "normal life". They were days when you could tell one day from another. On March 13, I met my friend Abir at the market. We had tea together in a fancy café. Its décor was so white that I had to request the waiter to dim the lights a little. Our conversation extended into dinner. I decided to cook mutton for us at home. My companion, Richa, returned from the office and joined us. There was some talk about the future. We named different cities. We wanted to escape the present and take shelter in another time. On the morning of March 16, our fifteen-year-old *Godrej* refrigerator exploded and died. In the evening, we went to Yusuf Sarai market to buy a new one. We found one that suited us best in Mohan Singh market instead. The timing of the whole event was uncanny. That evening I noticed a young woman on the sidewalk wearing a mask. It was a sign of the world to come. On March 17, we made a trip to the market close to home. I wore a black mask. The familiar attendant at Starbucks ushered us forward after aiming a temperature gun at our foreheads with a smile.

Such awkward moments are now part of our lives. Instead of laughing, people are fearful. As I walked out of the café to go home, I met my old student, Kimberley, a singer-performer. I asked what she was doing in the empty marketplace. She smiled and said she relished the emptiness.

New Dehli,
June 25, 2020

Newspapers, Plagues, Fish & Immortality

Monday, March 23

THE CHIEF MINISTER OF DELHI, THE MERCURIAL ARVIND KEJRIWAL, announced a complete lockdown of the capital city on Sunday night, from 6am today till March 31. On Sunday, heeding prime minister Narendra Modi's call, people all over the country observed "Janata Curfew" (a self-imposed curfew by the people, as suggested by the government) from morning till night. At 5pm, according to the prime minister's wishes, people came out on their balconies and verandas to clap and clang steel plates and other utensils as a mark of appreciation and gratitude towards those providing health services in fighting the spread of Covid-19. Religious connotations were attached to the shrill sounds that ripped the air. The sounds of clanging at the threshold of every household were supposed to drive away the evil spirits.

Astrological theories were aired on social media. In one case a famous actor in Hindi cinema proclaimed that 5pm on March 22 would herald the lunar phase of the new moon, and the vibrations from clapping and conch shells would drive away the evil virus and bacteria. It was a theory no physicist would dare offer. The actor thought his wisdom would endear him to the masses. But the fear of the virus was too real to be distracted by the lollipop of astrology. The star faced a huge backlash and deleted his piece of wisdom.

In India, we are living in a time of internal political war waged against people described as "anti-nationals", or enemies of the nation. The national enemy is either religious or ideological. The arrival of Covid-19 changed (and shook) the political discourse. The new enemy was not someone we could name, place, animalize or tame into a harmless thing. The enemy was not a poor, undocumented migrant or refugee. Nor was the enemy a terrorist carrying a Kalashnikov or AK47. The enemy this time was an invisible virus. No threat of violence, no new law, could intimidate the new enemy. Everyone was susceptible. We no longer faced the imaginary enemy carrying a real face. We faced a real enemy with no face. The enemy was neither religious nor ideological. The enemy was biological. Covid-19 won't discriminate between Hindus and Muslims, nationals and anti-nationals. The nation was forced to reconnect with the idea of "people".

I HAD SET an alarm for 6.30. Richa woke me up at 6.10. I set out for the vegetable store. When I reached the store, the man was surprised to see me. He had never seen me at that hour. But he understood why I was there early. The store was almost empty. I felt good to have woken up before the neighbourhood. People may have got enough in their homes already. The announcement of the lockdown by the prime minister at 8pm last night didn't bother them.

Vegetables and roots were laid out in large baskets all around the store: onions, tomatoes, potatoes, cauliflower, cabbage, beans, broccoli, carrot, beetroot, and more. They looked as fresh as the morning. Even though we had left the festival of Holi behind, summer was taking its time to arrive in Delhi. I realised I couldn't carry everything alone, so I called Richa to come and help me. We took enough to last us more than a week.

I was surprised to see the newspaper lying on the terrace. I had told the seller we did not need any more newspapers. I called to ask why he did not stop delivering it.

"Please sir, take it today. No newspaper from tomorrow," he said. I realised his situation. He would incur a loss he hadn't anticipated.

I imagined the coming days waking up to mornings without newspapers. We will read the news, but not on paper. Imagine if newspapers vanished one morning. The habit of reading news over a cup of tea in the morning becomes a thing of the past. Maybe that is when we will suddenly begin to remember our days with the newspaper.

DURING SCHOOL, I remember my passion for the *Telegraph* published in Calcutta (now Kolkata), because it was glossy and covered sports well. I was not adult enough for politics or editorials. Whenever I fell ill, I would request mother to go and get the paper from the neighbour's house. My father preferred the older *Amrita Bazar Patrika*. Much later, I learnt of other newspapers. You were supposed to read the *Statesman* for learning English. While reading, I realised the English was good but idiomatically very British. I was more at ease with the flowy, simple English. The *Times of India* had a good reputation. Dilip Padgaonkar was at the helm, as editor in chief. His front-page condemnation of the demolition of Babri Masjid (a sixteenth century mosque built in Ayodhya, on the orders of the first Mughal emperor, Babur) created ripples. It was a strongly worded piece that did not please my next-door uncle, who I thought was an enlightened man. He said, "These people can only condemn Hindus."

Six months later, in July 1993, Padgaonkar interviewed V.S. Naipaul at the writer's flat in London. Naipaul supported the demolition, saying "Indians are becoming alive to their history."[14] Which history? The history, Naipaul said, of the "great vandalising of India".[15] For him, all talk of "synthetic culture" portrays the mindset of "a defeated people".[16] Naipaul's vision of history is aroused by two things that have no connection with one another: the ruins of Hindu civilisation, and the vandalism that destroyed the Babri Masjid. Nostalgia is the chief culprit behind the modern fantasy of cultural revivalism. Naipaul was a parasite of history. He loved to feed on history's nightmares, lick its wounds, and offer us his parasitic wisdom. Naipaul treats history's latest nightmare as a panacea for the old. A keen-eyed writer, who has offered critical insights into the modern condition, Naipaul's sense of humanity was defeated by his sense of history.

Speaking of newspapers, I never took one during my nine years in a JNU (Jawaharlal Nehru University) hostel. I had stopped being a news person. I had no interest in the news around me. I was happy reading philosophy and literature. My friends thought it was important for a student of social sciences to read newspapers. They would ask me to give them one good reason against it. I did not have one. That is, until I read an interview with a poet (whose name I do not remember) in *World Literature Today*. He said he had stopped taking interest in history after the fall of Constantinople.

I laughed, as heads turned in the quiet reading room of the JNU library. But I had found my answer to future queries. I would say, I had no interest in India's postcolonial history, after the fall of Babri Masjid.

Friends ensured I did not miss things worth reading. Someone told me of Gabriel García Márquez's story that appeared in *Frontline*, reprinted from the *New York Times*, 'Shipwrecked on Dry Land.' It was about the tragic death of a young Mexican refugee boy, Elian, shipwrecked on the shores of America.[17] Someone said, "It read like a page torn from *One Hundred Years of Solitude*." Years later, discussing the article with students in my Literary Journalism class, I was nostalgic about my university days. Now I am nostalgic about the journalism class. The period of nostalgia is getting shorter. Either life is moving fast, or the world is changing faster.

Márquez's *Love in the Time of Cholera* was woven in the backdrop of a cholera epidemic. The book is set in a port city in Colombia in the late nineteenth century. If we have wild astrological theories on clapping and conch shells as a deterrent to the coronavirus, the unnamed city in Márquez's novel also had its local genius: 'From the time the cholera proclamation was issued, the local garrison shot a cannon from the fortress every quarter hour, day and night, in accordance with the local superstition that gunpowder purified the atmosphere.'[18]

The paradox unleashed by the epidemic was also apparent: 'The cholera was much more devastating to the black population, which was larger and poorer, but in reality, it had no regard for color or background.'[19] The effect of a pandemic — in an earlier time as now — is bound to reflect the class divide. Poor people living in congested areas, in poor economic and environmental conditions, will be prone to its spread and become affected. But the nature of the pandemic will still be equally threatening for everyone.

Márquez had spoken to Marlise Simons at the *New York Times* about his interest in plagues. There was an insomnia plague in *One Hundred Years of Solitude* that caused the death of birds. Márquez's words are insightful in the light of sudden lockdown. Sitting in Delhi, I read with horror and sadness the reports of the deaths rising in Italy and America. Doctors were taking risks to treat patients. But a new fear that was unknown to us, the fear of outside space — *agoraphobia* — had suddenly descended. It was hanging in the air.

I walked to the terrace in the afternoon but couldn't see any people. Everyone was indoors by the decree of fear. Only the vegetable vendor waited to take out his handcart. The breeze made the eucalyptus tree sway its leaves. It made me feel a little better. At least nature was moving.

In the interview, Márquez told Simons, "Plagues are like imponderable dangers that surprise people. They seem to have a quality of destiny. It's the phenomenon of death on a mass scale. What I find curious is that the great plagues have always produced great excesses. They make people want to live more. It's that almost metaphysical dimension that interests me."

The last two sentences struck me as insightful in relation to what we are experiencing right now. Thanatos intensifies Eros.

Soumya, a journalist friend from Delhi trapped in New York, said how in these extraordinary circumstances, she realised New York was not so much home, but "paraya mulk" (alien country). She was quarantined, and felt she had mild symptoms of the virus. She was worried about immortality: not leaving behind a book for the world to remember her by.

Another friend from India, a Muslim professor with roots in Hyderabad who teaches at a university in the US, told me she has immersed herself in writing a historical fiction on the life of a medieval princess. She was pained by the Islamophobia around her, among students and the public at large. She planned to live in the woods if things deteriorated further. Her decision is reminiscent of David Thoreau's *Walden; or, Life in the Woods*: a book and a lived project in the middle of nineteenth-century America, where nature is granted its place as the centre of life. Thoreau tries to find an economy of self-sustenance that fosters solitude, a retreat from the noise of modern civilisation, and a way to expand the horizons of solitude. He writes, 'I went to the woods because I wished to live deliberately, to front only the essential facts of life.'[20]

For the Muslim professor, the woods meant a retreat from hate, and the constant, tiring encounter with western prejudice. The West invented the "human being" in modernity but could never really incorporate "other people" into that idea. Meanwhile she plotted her escape through the novel. She was working on her immortality.

Milan Kundera commented in his novel, *Immortality*, 'Man reckons with immortality, and forgets to reckon with death.'[21] But Kundera forgot that life during an epidemic and similar situations makes people reckon with immortality *because* they are reckoning with death. The predicament of writers in our times is more aptly captured by what Jean-Pierre Melville (playing the fiction writer, Parvulesco) said in Jean-Luc Godard's 1960 film, *Breathless*. When asked in an interview, "What is your greatest ambition?" Melville says, "To become immortal, then die."

A play on the title of Márquez's book crept up on social media. 'Love in the Time of Corona' became a hashtag for difficulties faced by lovers due to the lockdown. The essence is perhaps best captured by twisting the title of a Quevedo poem: Love Constant during Plagues.[22]

It was a few minutes past 7 in the morning, right after returning with the vegetables, when I rushed to the ATM, only to discover my credit card wasn't in my wallet. I called Richa frantically. There was a momentary scare when she said she couldn't find the card. Everything quickly turns into an ominous sign in disturbing times. Finally, to my relief, she found it. After drawing out money I looked for an autorickshaw. I wanted to visit the fish market in the Bengali neighbourhood of Chittaranjan Park (or CR Park), and try my luck. CR Park was established in the 1960s for the displaced Bengali Hindu community, arriving from erstwhile East Pakistan. Its fish sellers are interesting people.

I was lucky to catch hold of an autorickshaw. The man had just dropped off four people and was willing to make any quick trip. He agreed to take me on double rates. I didn't mind. It was perfectly understandable under the circumstances. The road was empty, and he drove like a man racing against time. He needed to make as much money as he could before the police prevented him from plying his trade. Reaching the market, we found it was closed, except for one man looking at us. I went and asked him if he was selling fish. Yes, he said. I asked him when the market opens. It opens at 9am, he informed me. I asked him why he was there so early. He looked for an answer but didn't find one. I gave it to him, "You are here because I am here. I had to buy fish from you. It was ordained."

He smiled and told me the names of the fishes he had. I chose three different varieties. As he removed the scales and the fins, he asked, "Why do these Chinese eat bats and lizards? Can't they stick to tastier things like fish?"

I laughed, "Perhaps they get bored of the usual stuff, and love experimenting."

The man shook his head, "How can you be bored of fish?"

As I travelled back home in the auto, the words of the fish seller kept ringing in my head. I smiled to myself. My mind went back to that afternoon in JNU. My friend from the English Literature department, Ramesh Mallipeddi, said he would treat me to lunch at the library canteen. It was also called Gopalan's canteen. Gopalan was a mild, old, bespectacled man from Kerala. He charged us a pittance for a delicious plate of fish and chicken. In winters we would sit out in the sun and eat, looking into the forest. That summer afternoon, Ramesh and I were in the mood for fish. So, we ordered it, along with daal, vegetables and salad. Ramesh noticed I was engrossed in having the fish. He chose the perfect moment to say,

"God should have created only three things."

I looked up, momentarily distracted from my plate. He had my attention.

"What?" I asked.

Ramesh smiled and said, "Man, woman and fish."

We both laughed.

I was reminded of Günter Grass' *The Flounder*, a novel inspired by the German fairy tale written by the Brothers Grimm, 'The Fisherman and His Wife.' It was about women, food and war, and the narrative was interspersed with recipes that included fish.

The autowallah dropped me home. I paid him more than what we had agreed because he had waited for almost half an hour for the fish to be cleaned. He was anxious to find more passengers before having to vacate the streets. I wished him luck.

I had memorable times with autorickshaw drivers. When I left JNU and started living in a quiet locality in south Delhi, I still used to visit the university a lot. It was both home and the world for nine years. I missed it every day. I wanted to see how the sun fell on JNU, how the trees were doing, or to catch a familiar face walking past. The place slowly started growing unfamiliar. There were also invitations from friends to share a drink in the evening. On those occasions, I had my favourite autowallahs who would expect me in summer or winter nights outside the university's main gate. I did not have to direct them on my way home. When I submitted my doctoral thesis, I gifted them the two bottles of rum I had promised. I also gave one my audiocassettes as we had shifted to playing music on the computer.

The other autowallah I won't forget was the man who stood at the main road in Munirka. I was staying there briefly after passing out of JNU. The rent in Munirka is cheap, and you get regional variety in its small eating joints. A place full of surprises, it is also known for shady dealings.

One night I dropped off Richa, who I had been dating for a year, at her home in Karol Bagh. She recently joined Delhi University for a master's degree in English literature. It was late in the night in the thick of winter. We were looking for an autorickshaw when I saw his familiar face. As I bid Richa goodnight and she sat in the autorickshaw, the autowallah asked me if I was travelling with her as I usually did. I said no. He insisted on knowing why. I said we were saving money. He laughed and said I did not have to pay him for the return journey. I was surprised by the gesture. Karol Bagh was almost seventeen kilometres away. Seeing my hesitation, the autowallah laughed again and said, "Sing me Kishore Kumar songs on our way back."

He had heard me sing on trips before. I had found a fan. But truth is he did not want to deprive me of spending more time with my girlfriend. It was a gesture worthy of a modern folktale. Only people from small towns could write such stories in the forgotten nights of cities. What migrants bring to the city is what they find hard to receive: a gesture of love.

I dropped Richa outside her house and was happy to sing a few Kishore songs on my way back, to the memory of the night and the long and winding empty streets of Delhi.

Meanwhile, back home from CR Park through early morning unusually empty streets, I slept like a log for a long time. It took time for sleep to arrive. The errands of the morning exhausted me. Waking up early has always been a tough task. In the nine years in a hostel in JNU, the nights never ended, and the mornings never arrived. Only on Sundays, when the breakfast in the hostel mess was better than that served on weekdays, I would claim it despite the Saturday night hangover. Even the insipid coffee was special. The conversation in the mess made up for the coffee.

The most interesting person in the mess was undoubtedly Shakib bhai,[23] an older man who was finishing his doctoral degree. He was a Bengali Hindu, who had converted to Islam. He sported an unkempt beard and mostly wore kurta and pyjamas. Sometimes you would know he had taken a bath because the bottom of his trousers was wet. He spoke in Persian, but mostly to himself. While having tea, he would softly grumble and have serious and funny conversations that he alone enjoyed. He carried a butter knife, and for some strange reason would dip it in the glass while having tea or milk. Quite a character, he made us wonder and invent stories about him. One day I caught him talking while he was taking a bath. He was mumbling to himself. Passing, I heard him say, in Bengali,

"Mother, it all happened because of you."

One of the shortest and most enigmatic short stories that has stayed with me over the years is the Honduran born, Guatemalan writer, Augusto Monterroso's 'The Dinosaur': 'When he awoke, the dinosaur was still there.'

It evokes the return of prehistory, or the return of an extinct species from the Jurassic period, in the form of a dream. Shakib bhai's utterance has an oedipal ring to it. The idea of an original error, the error of origins, is an interesting one. I mention Monterroso to my Guyana-born historian friend, Anil Persaud. He reminds me of the shortest story of all, an unspeakably poignant story attributed to Ernest Hemingway: 'For sale: baby shoes, never worn.'[24]

When I woke up, Richa was there. Her reassuring presence makes waking up in the middle of a lockdown bearable. She smiles, and for a moment I forget about the virus, the scare, and the death toll rising in other countries. The pandemic is banging on India's door.

I cooked the "Tangra" (catfish) for lunch. Richa cut the vegetables. A simple recipe: sliced garlic, onions and tomatoes, put one after another in the pan after spattering cumin seeds in mustard oil. I only cook in mustard oil. I love its strong, pungent smell. I used turmeric and cumin powder. I also added green peas, and one potato sliced in small cubes so that it softens within minutes. I put the shallow-fried fish in the pan along with sliced ginger and green chillies, after pouring in water.

We never kept a cook. It is difficult to make domestic cooks (who are akin to helps) prepare cuisines to your satisfaction. Besides other issues, they are pressed for time. So I have been cooking myself at home all these years. But I would often get bored or tired. There was the delightful and easy option of eating at our favourite restaurants. But the lockdown meant no such luxury. I had to cook every day. I kept my spirits up for the task.

ON SUNDAY, MARCH 22, the women of Shaheen Bagh ended their iconic, street-side movement that had lasted over 100 days. They had gathered to protest the Citizenship Amendment Act, passed by the government on December 12, 2019. The Act was deemed exclusionary as it left out Muslims from the list of persecuted migrants offered asylum (and citizenship) in India.

The lockdown meant the highway protest had to be cleared off. But the women left the scene with a memorable gesture. They put their slippers on the empty beds they used in the protest.[25] In this way, they made their absence present, and produced a haunting image. It reminded me of the countless shoes kept outside the mosque before the men go in to pray. The shoes wait for their wearers, guarding themselves. In Shaheen Bagh however, the meaning is reversed. If the men leave behind their shoes before entering the sacred space of the mosque, the women leave behind their shoes as a mark of presence in their sacred site of protest. They won't allow anyone to think they have disappeared. The sacred at Shaheen Bagh was larger than faith. On January 12 this year, verses were read out from the Gita, the Quran, the Gurubani and the Bible. God was present in all names. Yet the empty shoes carried the weight of fragile life, a material sign of both persistence and vulnerability. Nothing could be more overwhelmingly human.

Of Children & Mothers in a Time of Forgetting

Tuesday, March 24

I WOKE UP LATE IN THE MORNING FROM UNEASY DREAMS.

The dream was full of snatches of childhood. The past is always nostalgic. But there is an acute longing that accompanies a dream about the past when you are facing a crisis in the present. The pandemic had forced my mind to swim back and recover what it remembered as something close to paradise. Paradise has been foolishly understood in history as a place for everyone. Each person has their own paradise, and yet it is a singularly impossible place to visit. Our dreams carry us to that place. It is pastoral because it is past. It is preindustrial, premodern, an escape from modern, urban life.

I lived in a town where people in the neighbourhood sometimes searched for cattle that hadn't returned. They asked, "Have you seen my cow?" I shook my head. They continued to search. To bring the animal home at dusk is a preoccupation, akin to looking for a lost child.

THE GARDEN OF Eden is the garden of childhood, where innocence and temptation live side by side. The erotic charge of temptation comes from its lure of innocence. Innocence is being inside an eggshell, a phase we gradually and reluctantly break out of. My paradise, idyll, or Garden of Eden, will always remain Shantiniketan, the university town where the poet, Rabindranath Tagore founded the Vishva-Bharati, with its green uneven meadows, tall trees, filtering sunlight, the myna bird, an occasional drove of donkeys, and so much silence that you must scream to know you exist.

During summer holidays, we would visit the family of my father's friend in Shantiniketan. While the elders were busy in conversation, or singing songs of Tagore, I would be playing in the meadow with their daughter who was a little older than me. We were barefoot like animals. We played hide-and-seek and catch-me-if-you-can. Flirtatious names for games designed for children. We were also on the swing, where 'with every lunge of the swing', I experienced 'the lunging pits' of feeling, just like in A.K. Ramanujan's poem, 'Looking for a Cousin on a Swing.'[26] Since then, I looked for her in every swing.

In *Immortality*, Kundera pondered the paradox of the childhood game of doctor. The little girl plays the patient, the little boy plays the doctor, and both play at being adults. As the boy examines the girl, their hearts beat harder. In *The Book of Laughter and Forgetting*, Kundera explores another aspect of childhood and paradise. Tamina, a woman who works in a café in Prague, travels to an island full of children. Here she realises that children do not live by the rules of privacy and individuality, nor the rules of decency. The experience turns to horror. An adult cannot return to childhood except by crossing the border.

I read these books much later, during my graduation, when they took me back to my time in the meadows of Shantiniketan and neighbourhood gardens. There is a Tagore song written in 1910 that captures the elusive moment. It is beautiful song, if translated badly in the *Gitanjali*. I offer my own translation:

'When I played with you, who knew what you were / Then there was no shame, no fear. Life flowed restlessly, as it were.'

Uneasy dreams are uneasy in any condition. But the difference hits you, after you wake up. Sometimes, even while dreaming, or after you have partly woken up, you may want to escape the world that awaits you a little longer and try to return to the dream. It is difficult to go back once you have opened your eyes. Like childhood and adulthood, there is a border between sleep and wakefulness. Once you cross it, you can't travel back.

I MAKE MY morning cup of Earl Grey tea. Except for the sound of the birds, which I don't mind, I write soundlessly for hours. I cannot hear the vegetable vendors cry out, as I usually do in the morning. The sudden lockdown must have made it difficult for vehicles carrying essential food items to cross interstate borders. It feels like a time of war. A world of adults having to rush indoors, like children.

Everyone was speculating on what the prime minister would say in his address to the nation at 8pm. He congratulated people for maintaining a self-imposed curfew. But in a grim tone he reiterated the need for further, and stricter, rules to combat the pandemic. He announced a nationwide lockdown of twenty-one days. The nation was under a three-week curfew. Ironically, it was not the prime minister who declared the emergency. Writers, journalists and doctors had already announced a medical and health emergency.

The PM said, "Forget what it is like stepping out of the house for twenty-one days."[27]

He implored the nation to forget.

You must forget the time you stepped out of your home. You must forget the footsteps of freedom. Delete the memory of the past. From now, you won't just miss the world, you will miss yourself. You will miss yourself in the world. But the world will also vanish. It will disappear into itself.

Pandemic-time is a frightening zone where you experience the forgetting of time.

In a rare gesture, the PM folded his hands while appealing to the people to stay at home. Normally, he would raise a finger as a challenge to the opposition that questions his rule. The haughtiness of the raised finger transformed into the humility of folded hands was a dramatic moment. The shifting stage of political theatre is dominated by a leader who raises his finger when he wishes to and folds his hands when it suits him.

As with everyone else, heads of state were being challenged in ways they could not have expected, in their case terms of resolve and intelligence.

I WAS WORRIED about my eighty-year-old mother, who lives in a Kolkata suburb. Living alone has made her impatient. She is absorbed in watching television serials and remains distracted when talking on the phone. She interrupts me, even when I am trying to share information about the pandemic and the lockdown.

My mother has developed a strange rule of perception over the last few years. If I try to explain any piece of news that warrants attention, she will appear confused and partly disinterested. She will understand the issue only after she hears it on television. She is better plugged into the TV than the world. The TV is her friend, philosopher and muse. Once I told her not to watch too many serials. She cut me off to say, "My children are all away, busy with their lives. The characters in the serial visit me every day. I learn about their lives. They keep me company. I can't do without them. Don't lecture me on what to do."

On a good day, I can win an argument with almost anyone. But even on my best day, I will lose to my mother. Her clinching statement has always been: "I have carried you for nine months. Don't try to teach me."

In Márquez's memoir, *Living to Tell the Tale*, he narrates how his mother comes looking for him, despite the knowledge that he is drinking with his writer friends. Before he can react upon seeing her, she says: "I am your mother."[28] It is confession and affirmation rolled into one. The primordial power behind that statement is unbeatable.

Mother handed the phone to the woman who helps to take care of her. I explain what they need to do and what they need to desist from doing in the present climate. I give her the background of the pandemic and its possible dangers. She listens patiently and assures me she will explain everything to mother and take care of things. It relieves me.

I get overwhelmed with guilt to have my mother stay by herself in her old age. But my education has divided us, our lifestyles. She knows that. "I lost my children in my desire to give them an English-medium education," she says with half regret.

Meanwhile, I get a text from Richa, visiting the nearby market. She tells me the place is shrouded in darkness and appears abandoned. A few days earlier we were seated in the café there, having tea. The waiter welcomed everyone with a yellow temperature gun, aimed at the forehead. It is ironic that, not too long ago, people were being screened for what they might carry *outside* their bodies. Now, even surveillance has turned biological.

She informs me that a dog sits on the dark veranda outside the ATM, whining. A dog's grief is difficult to understand because it lacks language. It is pure expression. I took that image as being representative of the crisis. The dog, "man's best friend," was clearly missing human company. It was missing attention. I found no comfort in the thought that our disappearance from the earth is registered in the eyes and whining of a dog.

Of Trees, the Forest & the Fox's Wedding

Wednesday, March 25

WOKE UP TO BIRD CALLS AND WONDERED WHERE I WAS.

I was happy to be among trees and birds after seven years of having lived in a one-room apartment that looked onto the ugly backside of other buildings.

The days were already slowing down. I was used to spending days and long hours at home. I occasionally taught an elective course on lyric poetry in the university and occupied myself with this for a time. Otherwise, I have been mostly writing. The lockdown did not shock me into a new life. As friend and writer, Amandeep Sandhu, wrote on his Facebook page on 18 March: 'For a writer, most days are quarantine.'

Since 2014, we have been witnessing the rise of majoritarian nationalism in India that predictably took a fascist turn. It was a nationalism against ourselves. I am reminded of Tagore's lectures on nationalism during World War I, published in 1917. He aired an aesthetic and moral disapproval of the 'the fierce self-idolatry of nation-worship'.[29] He thought 'nationalism is a cruel epidemic of evil'.[30] These observations were warnings.

My generation of Hindus grew up in the 1970s with Sikhs, Muslims and Christians together in school and in the neighbourhood. We did not need to learn diversity from textbooks.

We learnt it in our daily conversations, and on the football field. We did not *tolerate* difference. We were attracted to difference. It added flavour to the efforts of love and the quarrels of friendship. We grew up on good and crude doses of Hindi cinema. It fed us stereotypes, but they were funny and made us laugh. Unlike today's stereotypes that create monsters. What it gave us, above all else, was the beauty of Urdu poetry and popular music.

The transition from Indian to Hindu, from secular to religious, from the time of Jawaharlal Nehru to this time (post-2014), took sixty-seven years. Everything that we considered worthy of a democracy was now being undermined in the name of majoritarianism. Some people who lacked spines were cheerleaders for this change. They behaved like what Osip Mandelstam in another time and place called 'half-men'.[31]

THE WIND WAS blowing hard in the afternoon. It shook the doors of the house. I am always tempted by the wind to go out and feel its force. I have met others who feel the same. My old Meitei friend from JNU, Bidhan Laishram, told me of an afternoon like this, when he was a schoolboy in Manipur:

"We were having our summer vacation. Suddenly, the sky turned grey and a storm was brewing. The animals were rushing for shelter. Birds were flying back to their nests. I was standing at the doorstep, watching the scene when I felt a rush to go out. My mother saw me and understood what I was poised to do. 'Don't go out now. Look, even the animals are coming back,' she said, her voice drowned in the wind. I was in no mood to heed to any warning. I rushed out to feel the storm. I felt it was calling me out of my house."

The storm in nature had incited a strange storm within. The madness of nature invites us to release the madness hiding in our soul. My friend experienced that moment of release. When he narrated the story, I was reminded of the unforgettable episode, 'Sunshine through the Rain,' in Akira Kurosawa's *Dreams*. The sun is up, and it is still raining. A boy wants to go out, but his mother dissuades him, saying the foxes are having a wedding procession and they'll get angry if they see anyone. When I saw the episode, I was awestruck because I was told the same thing while growing up. Whenever it rained and the sun was up, I had not to venture into the garden and disturb the fox's wedding. I was surprised to learn that foxes, the most treacherous animal in folk tales (and the ones that make the stories exciting), had such a romantic side.

In Kurosawa's story, the boy heads out into the forest against his mother's warning. Youth is a time to throw caution to the wind. The boy is soon rewarded by the scene that unfolds: Foxes (*kitsune*) in human form walk through a smoky haze. The hollow, clicking sound of the music gives an eerie impression of a secret ritual. The wedding procession of the foxes looks very austere. The ambience anticipates lewd indulgence later. There are alert twists of the head as the foxes walk in a jerky rhythm, cautious to guard their mysterious ceremony. There is a suggestion of something sexually forbidding, particularly for human beings.

I WAS ON the terrace, enjoying the sway of the huge eucalyptus tree, its branches bent in all directions, having weathered many storms. We had been in this rented place for two years. Though

I liked many things about the house, I often said that I chose it because of the eucalyptus tree. It was the best neighbour I could ask for. I have grown up among trees in my hometown, Maligaon, near Guwahati, the capital of Assam. We had a garden. Maligaon means "The Gardener's Village". Every garden was looked after by the 'mali', or gardener, assigned once a week by the Department of Horticulture. Our gardener was a lively and sturdy man, Kishen Deo. I would watch him in the garden, making flowerbeds and preparing the soil to grow vegetables, using a trowel and a digging hoe. I learnt to use these tools under his supervision.

I missed having a garden of my own in Delhi. When I saw the eucalyptus, in my new rented place, I felt it stood for all the trees in my head, the trees I had lost. The tree was many trees. It stood for a forest of memory. We are children of a ruined garden. We are children of the memory of forests. A single tree resembles our broken ties with the forest.[32]

As we stole some time together on the dark terrace, I told Richa, "I can talk to this tree at night. I feel my ancestors live here. Even my old neighbours, long dead, I feel are here."

You can talk to trees in the oldest sense of communication. It is like talking to a grandfather, who does not speak, but simply listens to you with his grey, flowing beard, eyes closed. The Finnish poet, Paavo Haavikko, wrote:

So, be seated under the tree and listen to it,
Exchange pleasantries, talk to it.[33]

Trees encourage conversation by speaking the same way it

listens: silently. It helps us find the interlocutor within us. But trees whisper when there is breeze. It tells us things the world robs us of. The world of automobiles keeps us from hearing the tree and hearing ourselves. The automobile is deaf and turns us deaf. We model ourselves on the machine. There is an undetected madness in people who live their lives in the company of automobiles. Haavikko wrote:

> There are many wise men yet on the other hand
> Not a single case of madness among trees.[34]

Trees don't go insane because like wise men they can hear themselves.

I wanted to sit on the terrace and feel the wind. Since I had started writing this journal, it did not leave me much time to consider reading a book. I picked from the shelf the new copy of Milan Kundera's *The Book of Laughter and Forgetting* that I had bought from the last World Book Fair. Kundera was a major discovery upon my graduation. His novels from Faber & Faber were being reprinted in the early nineties in India by Rupa Publications. The first novel, *Immortality*, was priced at a mere Rs.60. I had bought it from the Guwahati Book Fair. The price meant a lot to a college student with peanuts for pocket money. I bought Kundera's remaining novels from Modern Book Depot, Panbazar, in Guwahati. Each time I saw a new title on the bookrack, I felt it had arrived for me alone. Encouraged by my mentor, Upal Deb, who taught English literature at the college where I studied political science, I reviewed Kundera's novels (*Immortality, The*

Unbearable Lightness of Being, The Book of Laughter and Forgetting and *Life is Elsewhere*) for the *Sentinel*, a local English daily. My father would take mother along to get the Sunday newspaper from a bookstore named D.B. Library, whenever my reviews made it into print. These were my first published pieces of writing and gave me the chance to meet D.N. Bezboruah, the magnetic chief editor of the newspaper. His scathing editorial on the ugly affair of local militants murdering a rural development activist, Sanjoy Ghosh, had created ripples. When a man who writes brilliantly is also brave, it adds to his charm.

The pages in my old copy of *The Book of Laughter and Forgetting* were falling apart. I sat down on a cane stool to read, experiencing a forgotten familiarity of the story. I did not have to read much to come across these lines that ring truer now, at least for us in India, than when Kundera wrote them:

> The assassination of Allende quickly covered over the memory of the Russian invasion of Bohemia, the bloody massacre in Bangladesh caused Allende to be forgotten, the din of war in the Sinai Desert drowned out the groans of Bangladesh, the massacres in Cambodia caused the Sinai to be forgotten, and so on, and on and on, until everyone has completely forgotten everything... Nowadays, time moves forward at a rapid pace.[35]

Kundera wrote of history galloping fast. I am thinking of the chain of events in India[36] just before the nationwide lockdown was announced. The lockdown brought new difficulties for the poor

Muslims who fled their homes during the Delhi riots and were living in relief centres.

News arrived of armed men of the Islamic State laying a six-hour siege of a Sikh religious complex in Kabul, killing twenty-five people. Covid-19 had already claimed fifty-eight victims in Afghanistan. The Islamic State is a malevolent political project that can't be cured by faith. It is among similar symptoms of modernity, where religion is reduced to brute territorial power.

BIRDS WERE RETURNING home. But godless men had lost the refuge in their soul.

I cooked mutton for dinner. Richa helped with cutting the vegetables. I kept the recipe simple again. I felt all meals under lockdown should be made light, in contrast to the heaviness of our solitude.

I splattered small cardamom, cloves and cinnamon in oil, then roughly sliced garlic and ginger, and onions. I placed in the pan the usual turmeric and spoonful of cumin and coriander powder. I followed it with tomatoes to add a tangy flavour to the masala. Then I put in the mutton and slow cooked, adding water later.

We Fear Bravely

Thursday, March 26

I WOKE A LITTLE EARLIER THAN USUAL AND SAT DOWN TO WRITE with my morning cup of tea. I decided not to read the news of the day, till I had written enough to feel a bit tired or distracted. I was already working on a book of political nonfiction when the lockdown was declared. I had to finish the whole manuscript by June and submit to my editor. The lockdown interrupted that project with an unanticipated but understandable force. It was not possible to avoid the news pouring in from the various corners of the world.

Everyone was suffocated by concern and anxiety, for themselves and for others. The fate of others would have a bearing on one's own fate. People around the world, connected by technology, were now connected by a deadly virus. We moved from the connectivity that facilitates conversation to the connectivity that facilitates death.

We boarded the train of progress. It took us through many exciting and dreadful places. Not only could we not think of getting off the train, it was not possible for us to do so. The surplus of goods made possible by technology had made us indulgent. Capitalism created an economy to sustain this indulgence. The idea of "choice" became supreme. To offer a reason for our choices was enough for them to be regarded necessary and important, even though they may be superficial and self-aggrandizing. The distinction between "good" and "bad" reason is still stuck on the superiority of argument alone. Rational arguments don't produce a social ethic based on care, love and justice. The idea of reason has ironically circumscribed our sense of choice. We have become the blind men of reason.

I recall the opening lines of 'Poetry for an Album', a poem by W.G. Sebald:

> Feelings my friend
> wrote Schumann
> are stars which guide us
> only when the sky is clear
> but reason is a
> magnetic needle
> driving our ship on
> till it shatters on the rocks.[37]

When the sky is murky, and thinking with feelings is difficult, we board the ship of reason, hoping it will sail us through. But reason hides its blindness from us. Its calculations always fall short of life, and reality.

Humankind wants to consume the world. Technology enables this. But just as a virus can infiltrate a computer and spoil — even destroy — the system, Covid-19 can enter the body and is transmitted by touch. We are porous computers.

I picked up a new book to read under the sun on the terrace. The Delhi sky looked clearer than ever. The blue was never so blue.

It was evident that a polluted city could have its clear air back when the automobiles were off the road for a while. The last time I had seen a bluer sky was probably in Srinagar, on a visit with a contingent of poets, in the winter of 2015.

The Delhi chief minister's odd-even rule (private vehicles with odd and even number plates being allowed to run on alternate days of the week) aimed at tackling the alarming rise in pollution was a scheme too little, too late. It helped ease the traffic but not pollution.

The book I decided to read was Fernando Pessoa's *The Book of Disquiet*, which I had bought from the World Book Fair in Delhi. A friend asked me years ago if I had read the book. I hadn't yet but intended to read it soon. He said, "If you finish that book, I won't speak to you."

What on earth did he mean? *Disquiet* is a fragmentary autobiography that Pessoa attributes to 'Bernardo Soares' (described as an assistant bookkeeper in Lisbon). Unlike a conventional autobiography, Pessoa/Soares describes a life partly unlived, giving us his difficult impressions about human existence.

It would be insensitive to consume the whole of it. It would be vulgar to consume the life of a man who had laid bare his smallest and almost impossible worries with such painful accuracy. But the point of reading a book is not to finish it. The truth is also the opposite: The book finishes you. It claims and kills your time on earth. Books like Pessoa's can never be finished.

The book begins with an introduction by William Boyd, who quotes three lines from 'Love is the Essential', a poem by Pessoa written in 1935, also the year of his death:

Man is not an animal
Is intelligent flesh
Although sometimes ill.[38]

Pessoa's precision is seen in all his work, but most sharply in the poet he called his master, Alberto Caeiro. I asked myself, reading those three lines: What does Pessoa seek to illuminate in comparing humans to animals? The animal mirrors the beast in us: wild, tame, instinctive, violent, scared, purposeful, and needing love. The metaphors of each of these aspects are spread among many animals. We share an analogical relationship with animals. They are our natural neighbours. They mirror our nature. Our flesh, however, is dictated by a special kind of intelligence. It has not only ensured our survival as a species, but also contributed to what is uniquely human: the invention of culture. The illness of the flesh is therefore not only natural but also cultural. Illness is a metaphor. For instance, desire — something we seek beyond ourselves — makes us ill.

Pessoa suffocates you with insights. He writes, that 'the prophets and the saints who walk this vacuous world, are exploited by God himself'.[39]

That is also the theme of *The Gospel According to Jesus Christ*, the great novel of the Portuguese Nobel Laureate, José Saramago. In a dramatic dialogue between God, Jesus and the devil at the end of the book, Jesus is shocked to discover that God was not interested in making evil disappear from earth. God's own power depended on the presence of the devil. Jesus realised God had tricked him to carry out his message on earth. He was a pawn in

God's plan to rule by any means, fair or unfair.

My reading was interrupted by the sight of two birds sitting on a branch of the eucalyptus tree. I had probably seen them earlier but did not have the time to pause and observe them. Vinod Kumar Shukla writes in a novel meant for the young and old alike:

> During childhood, we notice birds a lot. As we grow up, we keep noticing less.
>
> We speak while sitting. We mumble to ourselves. We even speak in our dreams. We speak lying down. But the bird of colourful feathers, speaks only when it flies. If it sits, it goes silent.[40]

The lockdown has returned us to our lost childhood. It has returned us to birds. It has returned us to ourselves.

The two pretty birds sitting on the same branch seem to be lovebirds. Birds don't grow up with families. They don't have to convince other birds about the partner they choose. They can fly around happily with the one they love. This speaks of a more hassle-free life. It helps to have wings. I snapped a picture of them on my phone and sent it to "Bird Man". He lived as a "PIG" in JNU's Jhelum hostel. PIG is an affectionately blunt term for Permanent Illegal Guest.

Bird Man replied promptly: Yellow-footed green pigeons, "Hariyal" in Hindi.

CAMUS IN *The Plague* tells us:
'(E)ach of us has the plague within him; no one, no one on

earth is free from it. And I know, too, that we must keep endless watch on ourselves...'[41]

We have become watchmen, standing guard at ourselves, at our shadows. We terrorise ourselves with caution. We become extremely careful about what we touch, and if we touch, we immediately wash our hands with soap for at least twenty seconds. We are mindful of the merest hint of a sore throat, or rising temperature. We also have the time now to watch others, and not just the human species. We carry the virus in our heads, in our sleep, and some with intense paranoia, perhaps even in their dreams. Fear is our only mode of retaliation. We are brave, we fear bravely. We cannot laugh at ourselves. The absurdity of survival must be taken seriously.

Meanwhile deaths from Covid-19 were rising alarmingly. Someone with a dark and untimely sense of humour likened the global death toll statistics to an Olympic games medal tally. Italy more than doubled the number of deaths in China, where the pandemic was said to have originated. Even Spain had edged out China. France crossed 1,000. The US was approaching 1,000. Iran crossed 2,000. When death becomes a statistic, morality turns utilitarian: maximize benefits for the greater number. Doctors were fighting the hardest, not just to recover infected patients, but to not become infected. Unlike the God of religion, doctors have real and difficult responsibilities. Saving lives during a catastrophe is not just a heroic endeavour in the time of a medical emergency but also a moral emergency.

Someone wrote on Twitter this afternoon: 'Always knew my true purpose was lying on bed the whole day to save humanity.'

It is no joke that it is time to rediscover leisure, the pleasure of doing nothing.

One of Pessoa's heteronyms, Álvaro de Campos, has a poem written in 1928, 'Deferral,' about procrastination. I had read out the poem in a workshop on anti-work by old world anarchists years ago. The poem begins:

> I'll spend tomorrow thinking about the day after tomorrow,
> And then maybe, we'll see; but not today...,
> Today is out of the question; today I can't.[42]

The postponement of work, the refusal to be productive, is also a critique of the demands of capitalism, and modern life. Campos writes of the 'anticipated and infinite weariness, / A multi-world weariness just to catch a streetcar'.[43]

The poet feels like a tired automobile. He realises he's had enough of being the everyday machine, driven around by the demands of work against his wishes (the wishes of his leisure, his pleasure). Each act opens worlds of meanings, possibilities. Campos had enough, indulging in multiple gestures and manoeuvres to make life happen. He has realised, the only way out of the trap of modern life is to simply refuse to move, to postpone the act of thinking until tomorrow.

RICHA LOVES AND learns contemporary dance. Tonight, she started taking her few online Gaga dance classes, mostly on New York time. The contribution fee for these classes was meant to support independent artists who were out of work. I asked Richa, how different was the experience of taking part in a dance class conducted online. She missed the energy she feels from having fellow dancers in the same room. But it was replaced by a sense of being part of a universe of solitudes, where over 600 dancers across the world were participating from their individual spaces.

Covid-19 has added a new and unexpected value to the act of leisure. Of course, only the privileged can afford it. You are free to feel guilty. I am cooking almost every day, washing the dishes, and writing this book. I also get time to daydream and scrutinize the past.

The Disease Arrived via Aeroplanes

Friday, March 27

News of the mass exodus of migrant workers slowly began to emerge.

On the night of 25 March, after the PM spoke to the nation, around 2,000 daily wage workers from Ahmedabad walked for hours without food and water to reach their hometown in Rajasthan's Bichhiwara tehsil. Once they reached the Rajasthan border, some of them were put on trucks. Bhole Kumar, who worked as a mason on construction sites, walked 170 kilometres from Noida to a place near Meerut. He told a journalist, "Hawai jahanzon se bimari ayi hai. Hum to laye nahi. Par sadak pe bhooke hum ghoom rahe hain."[44] ("The disease arrived via aeroplanes. We did not bring it. But it is we who are roaming the streets, hungry.")

The lockdown was timed to avoid escalation of the pandemic. It was a logical necessity. The poor are not high on the government's agenda but rather an afterthought. It is always a little late, always too late, to address the poor.

There was panic behind the decision. The prime minister never looked as rattled as he did now. The pandemic did not only put people at a disadvantage, but political regimes as well. The regime must suddenly take care of everybody because the virus won't spare anybody. The impact of the government's hasty decision created a ripple effect in the daily wage workers, who suddenly began to flee to their native villages and towns.

It was mad to have a single decision for two classes that lived by completely different economies. A lockdown introduced different problems for different classes of people. The middle class and elite could buy their essentials and scramble home. For the migrant workers, home was far away and essentials nowhere in sight. They were fleeing not the virus, but the lockdown. They heard of the virus. But starvation was a more urgent concern. With work shut down, came fear. With food stores closing, the workers had no option but to leave. There were no concrete, official assurances regarding food supplies. Bhole Kumar's statement was ironic, but its implications were tragic. The labouring class suffered for no fault of its own. It was the class that knew luxury that had brought the virus from elsewhere. The logic was unjust.

IN THE AFTERNOON, Richa met Menoka, my Bengali neighbour, on the terrace, and learnt of her predicament. Menoka is an engineer, and lives with her mother and young daughter. Her husband lives in Paris. She was desperately missing her cigarettes. The essential goods of addiction weren't part of essential services. Those who hadn't stocked up enough alcohol were worried too. The sudden slowness of time was difficult to sail through without a high. Each day was a slow hangover.

Menoka turned to the garbageman and others to help persuade a cigarette shop owner to bail her out. She bought six packets at twice the usual price. She had to pay for a favour. Menoka loves two things: cigarettes, and her plants — both foliage and flower plants — that she has carefully chosen and keeps in earthen pots in her balcony and terrace.

Menoka also shared a story about her chauffeur, Salim, who lived in another part of Delhi. He was caught by the police while on his way to draw money from the ATM. The police took away his 'Aadhaar card' and promised they would return it later. The law can pressure you and make life uncomfortable. You should think yourself lucky it doesn't cause physical harm, and count its gentle disfavours as a blessing.

I COOKED ROHU fish curry for lunch. I used the same recipe as I did for "Tangra" except that I added small slices of onion flower stock ("Peyajkoli" in Bengali, often wrongly translated as spring onion or scallion). It turned out well.

REPORTS POURED IN of police heavy-handedness towards journalists, delivery boys helping with essential services, and even doctors. Police made citizens perform sit ups, and crawl on all fours. Some faced the baton. You won't catch a policeman laughing while doling out discipline and punishment. But he reminds you of the school or neighbourhood bully. Be it the doorkeeper guarding the law in Kafka's parable, or the policeman guarding the streets during lockdown, power experiences immense pleasure in being obstinate and an obstacle to someone.

These assaults are a consequence of the state machinery that encourages the police to come down hard on anyone who appears to defy the government's orders. The protest against the passing of the new citizenship law has created a tense and antagonistic relationship between police and citizen. It appears the police have lost the state of mind to distinguish between protest, healthcare and essential services.

The saddest news of the day was the Eidgah camp in northeast Delhi's Old Mustafabad, meant for Delhi's riot victims, being shut down by the authorities. People whose houses were burnt, and their savings stolen, would now be without shelter.

Mrs. Dalloway's Flowers & the Grass at Purana Qila

Saturday, March 28

I WOKE UP LATE MORNING. JUST IN TIME TO CATCH THE CRY OF THE vegetable vendor. It was a sudden, welcome reminder of the earlier life. The vendor's voice sounded unreal, as if from another time. Did we switch back to the past? Or was the past restored?

This was not the past of *Remembrance of Things Past*, but the past we know as the everyday. When it exists, we often don't even notice it. We take the everyday for granted. The history of the everyday, as Gandhi said, is never written. We don't write the history of harmony. We write of history with a capital H, the history of strife. The history of the everyday is the history of a time that exists in the blurry lines between memory and forgetting. The days we remember are days of events, personal, social, or political.

I walked to my terrace to see the vendor. His handcart was full of fresh vegetables. The tomatoes were ripe. But I had enough to last me a few days more. I was simply happy to see him, glad he was back to his routine and daily earning. He wore a mask. It muffled his voice when he announced his presence in the neighbourhood. It was a necessary hazard to prevent a more serious one.

After sitting down with my tea, I checked WhatsApp. A journalist friend in Hyderabad, Kakoli, uploaded a picture of flowers, a vine with small, red clusters she found on her way to the grocery. I asked her what flowers they were. "Madhabi Lata," she said, taking the Bengali name. It is also called the Rangoon creeper or the Chinese honeysuckle.

Flowers take different names in different countries and languages. Strangely, I developed an interest in flowers through my father. I say strangely, because my father did not have an eye or ear for aesthetics — music, cinema, or literature. But he had a keen eye for flowers. Fathers are strange creatures. My father was an employee at Northeast Frontier Railway and would often go on official duty to north Bengal and the nearby hills. He brought rare flowers from these places, unavailable in our hometown. The flowers were the envy of neighbours and passersby. My favourite was the Magnolia. Just one Magnolia in full bloom could rival the moon. When the moonlight fell over it, it lit up the heart of darkness. Another favourite of father (and mine too) was the legendary Ashoka flower. It bloomed in clusters of thin red stem-like petals, with dark green leaves. The Buddha, it is believed, was born under the Ashoka tree. Ravan, the legendary king of Lanka in the Sanskrit epic the *Ramayana*, had kept Ram's consort, Sita, in the "Ashok Vatika", or the Ashoka forest. Even though the scientific name Saraca Asoka means "sorrowless", the flower is associated with fertility and amorous feelings.

I wondered if Kakoli would have paused on earlier occasions to take such a picture and post it, despite her love of flowers. The lockdown slowed things down and made us pause over the little things of beauty we might otherwise hurry past on busy days. The presence of these flowers was a metaphor for a life she had left behind. Trapped behind walls, we become sensitive to each thing of beauty in the outside world deserving of our attention.

VIRGINIA WOOLF'S 1925 novel, *Mrs. Dalloway*, is the story of a woman in postwar London who recovers from influenza. (Woolf was witness to the same flu pandemic in early twentieth-century England that the Hindi poet and writer, Suryakant Tripathi — better known by his nom de plume, Nirala — faced in India, and wrote of the devastation it caused in his life.[45]) Woolf's protagonist, Clarissa Dalloway, returning to life like the rest of the town, has a thing for flowers. The novel begins with the famous line, 'Mrs. Dalloway said she would buy the flowers herself.'[46]

She goes to the florist — Mulberry's — on Bond Street, and discovers 'delphiniums, sweet peas, bunches of lilac... masses of carnations'[47] and roses. She chooses her flowers, moving 'from jar to jar', and 'this beauty, this scent, this colour'[48] passes over her like a wave. Dalloway is rejuvenated by flowers. Flowers here are not a metaphor of recovery from illness but a sign of recovery. They represent the sensual delight of life.

Woolf's essay 'On Being Ill',[49] published a year later in 1926, begins with how illness, including the pandemic of influenza, exposes on the one hand 'the wastes and deserts of the soul', as much as the 'precipices and lawns sprinkled with bright flowers'.[50]

Flowers emerge as an image of bounty and delight during good health. Woolf finds in illness a time to reflect on nature to learn endurance. She speaks of the stillness of flowers: the rose with its 'demeanour of perfect dignity and self-possession'.[51] Woolf reminds us, 'poets have found religion in nature; people live in the country to learn virtue from plants.'[52] It is then, a double-learning: Flowers are reminders of the colour of life, and of an essential stoicism. Flowers are beautiful and ascetic: A Woolf-ish paradox regarding the aloofness of beauty. Perhaps Woolf is mirroring herself through this natural description.

I KEPT WRITING, and soon it was afternoon and time for lunch. Richa boiled broccoli and carrots. After boiling the vegetables, she added raw onions, used olive oil for dressing, and squeezed lemon on top. It was good to have with eggs and vegetables.

I received an email from a student. I was invited to co-teach the lyric poetry course at Ambedkar University. I loved teaching so long as I had time to write, which is why I had not joined full time. This semester, I replaced Baudelaire, Akhmatova and Octavio Paz with fresh names: Ilya Kaminsky and Najwan Darwish. I wanted to discuss contemporary poets who wrote innovatively against power. I retained the Kashmiri-American poet, Agha Shahid Ali. In his piercing and delicate voice we hear the beauty and sadness of Kashmir.

I had taken the students to Purana Qila (Old Fort) for a class. I could not believe that this exceptional day was less than a month ago. The trip to a medieval garden in the city appeared now to be a dream. There is a suddenness about how a nightmare may suddenly descend upon people's lives and render the ordinariness of the immediate past exceptional.

That day at Purana Qila, sitting on the grass, we discussed poets. A dog was lying beside us and listened attentively. Later, we read Agha Shahid Ali's *The Walled City: 7 Poems on Delhi*. Some lines catch you by the throat:

> The Two-Nation Theory is dead
> But the old don't forget.
> In this city of refugees,
> trains move like ghosts.
> The old don't forget.[53]

There is no refuge in memory, only the same old noise of blood. Yet people hold onto the memory of strife to create new wedges in the present. Memory is a record book of errors.

I read out a couple of my own poems. Students loved my poem on the Kamakhya Temple. They said, "It's the best we read today."

I felt happy about the compliment. I wrote the poem from memory, almost two decades after I left my hometown for good. I wrote remembering the little details from many visits to the temple. It is a poem of return to a place that I never returned to. When a place in memory returns on the page, it does so with a rare intensity.

I am also fascinated by this unexpected moment of encounter: the memory of a temple, sitting with students in Purana Qila. It reminded me of the poem where the late Palestinian poet, Mahmoud Darwish, recalled his meeting with Yannis Ritsos in Athens, while he visited Pablo Neruda's house on the Pacific coast.[54] Here's my poem, dedicated to a double-memory.

Manash Firaq Bhattacharjee

KAMAKHYA

Spiral roads take you up
An occulted hill
The glacial river flows by,
Your spiralling eyes
Are full of green water,
You breathe
A vertiginous air,
Trees laden with monkeys
Greet you anciently,
You hear bells
Tolling against bad spirits
Sinisterly pious –
Priests, sheep
Vie for attention,
Flowers are food, mantras
Money,
You remove your shoes
Walk on old stones
They erase your presence
You are footsteps
With eyes of forgetting,
Divinities on walls
Pose — to stall your path
Tempt you,
Their bodies, counsels
On stone –

The Town Slowly Empties

Telling you, go break
The stones in your body
Become body
Spread your organs,
Branch out like flowers
Flower, branch,
Go, turn into verbs
Look, beside you
Goats are slaughtered
They wait, then –
Executed by a syllable
Their blood
Is our feast, we feast
On death,
Our mother bleeds –
To birth us,
Blood is birth, death
Regeneration
Kamakhya,
Dark spring,
Invites us below –
We go with careful steps
Where it bleeds
Water,
Blood is water,
On our forehead of water
A mark of blood,
It marks our fate,

Fate, marked by return
To roots
Of vanished, deserted
Homes,
Where we were born,
Will never die,
We die elsewhere,
Without roots
We are homeless figs
In the pyre,
In a fit you see –
Temple walls
Hoisted by pigeons,
Why do birds
Die clinging to walls,
What attracts
Feathers to stones,
No one knows
Inside the garbhagriha
Dark rumbles,
You go inside your head
Deeper, down,
Walled by fear, desire,
Touch the yoni
Waiting since ages
To remind you
Where you come from,
Kamakhya,

The orifice of origins,
Performs a ritual
Of blood's regenerative
Cycles,
Man sacrifices his animal –
For he lacks the blood
Of a woman,
Goats are muted spectators
Of self-annihilation
Or of delirium,
Of what man cannot hold –
In Kamakhya,
Stones bleed myths

My student, Priyanka Sahu, wrote to say that the 'trip to Purana Qila in the name of poetry was something pending in my history of education'. Poetry is better inhaled in open air. We are grateful to the Mughals who left us wonderful gardens, where we can steal time from within the city. Time revolves differently in the architecture of these gardens. Priyanka also sent me an inspired poem of her experience. She wrote of the 'stark greenery that mocks you / with a blinding hue of colour /... the smell of freshly mowed grass'. I shared with her a poem by another student from an earlier group that I had taken to Purana Qila. That poem had the line, 'I sit, devoid of footwear, allowing the touch of grass.'

When city dwellers get a touch of grass, the encounter leaves behind a sensuous residue of experience that translates into language. Words like "smell" and "touch" are naturally evoked.

Nature evokes nature. In his paean to grass, Walt Whitman was aware:

> That when I recline on the grass I do not catch any disease,
> Though probably every spear of grass rises out of what was once
> catching disease.[55]

The fresh spring of grass is a sign of life, tied to the soil and time (disease). We barely escape a brush with nature's illness, to enjoy the grass. In Jayanta Mahapatra's poignant and meditative poem, 'The Abandoned British Cemetery at Balasore, India,' he gives us his encounter with a remnant of colonial history. He meets the 'forgotten dead'[56] of thirty-nine British graves, with names inscribed upon them. Some, or all, had died in the cholera pandemic of 1817–1824. Mahapatra writes:

> Of what concern to me is a vanished empire?
> Or the conquest of my ancestors' timeless ennui?
> It is the dying young who have the power to show
> what the heart will hide, the grass shows no more.
>
> Who watches now in the dark near the dead wall?
> The tribe of grass in the cracks of my eyes?
> It is the cholera still, death's sickly trickle,
> that plagues the sleepy shacks beyond this hump of earth.[57]

The poet caught between two dead histories, the colonizer's

and his own people, finds no solace in the signs of life — 'the grass' — that lies around him. The dead teenagers — the nineteen-year-old wife of a captain, and a seventeen-year-old daughter — reveal his heart's regret more intensely. The shadow of the plague has covered the place and the spirit of hope. Mahapatra is confronted by hopelessness. Even the greenness of grass fails to stir him.

MEANWHILE MORE REPORTS poured in of the unfolding crisis on Delhi's borders. Migrant workers were fleeing the city out of fear and hunger. Ram Bhajan Nisar, a painter among them, set out on foot with his family of three, a wife and two children. He asked, "How can we eat if we don't earn?"[58] His family could hold on for four or five days but did not have enough beyond that.

Nisar's question stares us in the face. He, and labourers like him, live on a minimal level of subsistence. Any slackening of daily earnings takes them closer to the possibility of going without food. The fragile economy of their lives keeps them barely alive. It is the failure of the welfare state to provide a security net for the working class. Their lives go unprotected.

If the farmer grows our crops, if workers from factories produce our goods, migrant workers construct our cities. They relay bricks and cement from one person to another, over hours. Slowly, over days, the building takes shape. The workers occupy the building till the last job is done. When the building is ready, it is time for them to leave. Their traces vanish from the building. The occupants arrive to lay claim. Months of labour are forgotten. The memories of labour that make our lives possible, that build our homes, are not part of our memory.

Migrant workers took off on foot from various parts of the country to their hometowns in Bihar, Uttar Pradesh, Rajasthan, and Jharkhand. They were hoping for buses provided by the state but did not want to waste time waiting. The Delhi chief minister tried to persuade workers not to leave. He promised food and shelter. It was not enough assurance, and evidently too late. Workers trust what they see, and not what they hear. Their lives are too exposed to uncertainty to trust the insincerity of politics.

IN THE FAMINE of 1784, the Nawab of Awadh, Asaf-ud-Daula, came up with an extraordinary resolution: People who helped to build the grand mosque, Bara Imambara, will be provided with food. The double-economy of this grand initiative yielded historic results. Legend has it, the famous mutton pulao, originally a peasant dish, became a royal dish of the Nawabs who discovered it during an inspection of work at the Imambara. The technique of "dum pukht" (slow cooking and steaming of the meat, spices and other ingredients over a low flame, in a pot sealed with dough) is used to make this aromatic pulao.

In feudal times, a Nawab found a way to address the problem of hunger during famine. But in a democracy, you have a government that has failed to anticipate or address a similar problem during a pandemic.

Copper Coins & Abstract Shit

Sunday, March 29

I THOUGHT OF READING ZBIGNIEW HERBERT TODAY. HE WAS among the best postwar Polish poets. Herbert's rise as a poet coincided with the decline of the Stalinist hold on Polish culture and literature. Herbert had good reasons to dislike communism for what it did to his country. I took out his book of collected poems. I love the black and white cover, with Herbert lighting a cigarette. I prepared tea and checked the news.

The fragile peace was broken. Thousands of migrant workers had gathered in Delhi's Anand Vihar bus station, hoping to find a bus that would take them home. Some had heard of a dangerous virus putting lives in peril. But all they were certain of so far was the threat of hunger. They were also scared of the police.

The Delhi chief minister had promised distribution of food, but it was not enough. Staying in the city was difficult without being able to pay the rent. With work suspended indefinitely, there was no other option for these daily wage earners but to head home. There were four-year-olds on their fathers' shoulders, and ninety-year-olds with walking sticks.

When the prime minister declared the lockdown on March 27, the decision was superficially meant for everyone. *Politically*, it was meant for the middle class and elite alone. The poor live outside the government's thinking. In normal circumstances, while everyone else is working toward a better life, the poor work against hunger. If emergency for the elite meant social alienation with immediate effect, for the migrant workers it meant social chaos. The state of emergency pushed the poor (closer) to hunger.

I could not open the pages of Herbert until after lunch. A cool breeze was blowing, and the sun was gently warm. I took my cane stool and sat with my back to the sun. Herbert's poems speak of a man who has quietly observed life from the margins, his observations of the sea a natural metaphor for life. There is similarity with his Polish counterpart, Czeslaw Milosz, which isn't surprising. But Herbert is darker, and sharper. It is rare to decipher a smoky voice in poetry (the way you can describe a singer having a smoky voice). Herbert's voice is like that, but it doesn't lack precision. Let me share these powerful lines from the poem, 'WALL':

'We stand against the wall. Our youth has been taken from us like a condemned man's shirt. We wait. Before the fat bullet lodges itself in our necks, ten or twenty years pass.'[59]

I was reminded of the film on Kashmir, *Haider*, by Vishal Bharadwaj (based on the script by Kashmiri writer, journalist and friend Basharat Peer). In one scene, we hear the shrieks of young men in custody, piercing the silence of the night. The heaviness is on screen, and one shudders to imagine how it would be in reality.[60]

I am also reminded of Yannis Ritsos' *Diaries of Exile*, where he recounts long and difficult hours in prison. I plan to reread the book soon.

It is strange to associate youth with the time of waiting,

because the time of youth is activity. But political activity is risky, and might put you out of the sun, or the sun out of you. In her historic poem, 'Requiem' (1961–63), Anna Akhmatova describes how she stood among patient, old mothers for 'seventeen months in prison queues in Leningrad'.[61] They were waiting for the release of their young sons who were imprisoned on flimsy grounds by Nicholai Yezhov, the secret police official under Stalin. In a remarkable lyric poem of witnessing and resilience, Akhmatova registers her presence 'here, where I stood for three hundred hours / And where they never, never opened the doors for me.'[62]

I SPEND AN hour or so cooking and washing dishes. I cooked mutton in mint leaves for lunch. I grind mint and coriander leaves with green chillies and add it to the sauce that contains masala, garlic, ginger, onions and tomatoes. I add a cup of curd.

I prefer less spice these days. Once upon a time, I used to have whisky with stuffed red chilli pickle made in Andhra Pradesh. I have enjoyed pork with the famous "raja mirch" (or king chilli), made in Meitei, Naga and Khasi styles. A roasted form of the king chilli is also used in the special chutney made with fermented fish. Red chilli was brought to India by the Portuguese in the early sixteenth century. Before them in Mughlai cuisine black pepper was used.

During lockdown, I miss meeting the waiters from the nearby market. I miss speaking to Jerry, the young Malayali food enthusiast and manager at the restaurant, Fig & Maple. I would have long conversations with him about food, alcohol, and the hazards of majoritarian politics. He introduced me to the delicacy of Kollam fish curry, made with mustard paste and curry leaves, and served with yellow rice. He and his girlfriend considered the World Book Fair in Delhi every January a "pilgrimage" and saved up money for it.

I took time to speak Bengali with the young male waiters in Carnatic Café. I usually hide my Bengali identity in public. It probably comes from a sense of estrangement with my community which I seek to retain. It also helps me practice my little mischief: eavesdropping on Bengalis bitching about other people.

I don't want to be the universal man. But I also don't want to be Bengali.

Rimbaud stated in a letter written in 1871 to his friend, the poet Paul Demeny: 'I is another' (*Je est un autre*).[63] The self cannot be defined because the self is always seeking to be someone else, someone it is not. You can't recognise the self through conventional markers of identity and rational knowledge.

The most radical exemplar of Rimbaud's declaration, for someone who is alienated from his community, is Melvin,[64] the young man from Nagaland at a nearby café. When I chatted with him for the first time, I tried to impress him with talk of pork and the king chilli. He looked unimpressed. I told him the recipe of pork I had invented and named, "Halfway Goa" (marinade the pork Goan style, in lime juice and roasted and crushed mustard seeds, before cooking the meat in the northeast way, in its own oil, with crushed garlic and ginger, onion slices, tomatoes, masalas, and kaffir leaves). Melvin listened patiently, but there was a strange discomfort on his face. I was deeply puzzled. I couldn't imagine what was wrong until he explained. I listened in amazement: He ran away from home because spices did not suit his palette. He looked for a job in a city where people were not mad about spicy food. Someone told him Delhi, and so he ended up here. The only meat he liked was chicken. Otherwise, he was happy being vegetarian. I was incredulous. If I told this story to anyone, they wouldn't believe me. But truth is stranger than fiction.

I could not be friends with Melvin on matters of food. But I succeeded in something neither of us anticipated. I don't remember what prompted it, but one evening I was telling him about my schooldays. I mentioned how I often wrote letters to my girlfriend and became so adept at letter writing that other boys would come to me to write letters for them. They would tell me their feelings and I would turn them into a bouquet of words. The role of the surrogate writer of love letters helped me to better understand my own feelings. It also improved my felicity in the English language. Sometimes boys are insincere and exaggerate their feelings to the point of using someone else's words to pass off as their own.

My story had a great effect on Melvin. He smiled and shook his head in disbelief. He too wrote letters to a boy in his schooldays, he said shyly. It was clearly a cherished part of his memory.

The need to write to someone early in life to express one's feelings is an introduction to the aesthetic condition of modern life. Letters become emails and emails become chats and text messages. Language grows more and more pinched. The literary becomes literal. The mask of culture is torn off to reveal its skeleton. The new technology of love is an abbreviation.

I miss Melvin's smile, and Jerry's enthusiasm regarding cuisines. I have no idea when I will see them again. They were next door, in the nearby market. It is doubly strange because I haven't left for another city or part of the world. But today they appear remote. As if a huge wave suddenly appeared and separated us.

MEANWHILE, I AM engrossed in writing this book. I still have time to while away, stare into the blue horizon, and do nothing.

What does this lockdown do to time, at least our time, the privileged lot?

The most vulgar idea of time that capitalist society threw at us is caught in the popular saying, "Time is money." It means so many things at once: Time outside money is empty of content, or meaningless. Time makes sense only when you are putting in hours at work, when you are being productive. Time is something you earn, daily, hourly. Time is measurable, and earnable. You can count time. Time is in your hands. Your banknotes are your time. You sacrifice time to earn what you spend for a better life. Time is not your own.

What about life? Is the meaning of life to be solely derived from the ability to be productive and earning a livelihood? Does life 'count' for anything beyond the time spent in work? Octavio Paz writes in his long poem, *Sunstone*:

> better to be stoned in the plaza than to turn
> the mill that squeezes out the juice of life,
> that turns eternity into empty hours,
> minutes into prisons, and time into
> copper coins and abstract shit.[65]

That is precisely our condition. Not just the condition we are in after the declaration of the nationwide lockdown, but our condition even before the catastrophe.

Having avoided a full time profession, I tried to devote my time to creative work, as well as in reading and contemplation. I kept clear of the calculating (and calculative) hands of the capitalist clock. I wanted to live outside that time and be closer to a life where time is not tick-tocking on my wrist. I sought the world instead, looking for company over tea or coffee or wine. Often I would hear, "I am busy today/this week…" Time stood like a wall between us. I paid the price of not being busy, in a busy world.

I am busy. This declaration grants an existential superiority to the person uttering it. It is possible the busy person is unhappy rather than pleased about being busy. But she excuses herself, leaving you to deal with your desire for company alone. You fall outside the sphere of productive time. You feel like an animal living the bare life of someone who is free.

Karl Marx's idea of 'alienation'[66] is limited to the condition of labour. Max Weber's idea of 'disenchantment'[67] addresses the larger problem of the rationalization of life. Both touch upon the structures of work and social relations in modernity. Life has been emptied of what Paz calls 'juice', the wellspring of spontaneity. Life has been reduced to abstract shit.

When asked how she was doing, my mother would often use the Bengali phrase, "We don't have a life." What she meant was the daily drudgery of life, the routine of office and household work. Life was elsewhere. Life was always a little further away. Life was a bird sitting on the branch of tomorrow, waiting to take flight.

Richa took an hour's online class of Afro Flow Yoga, taught by an American artist. I felt it was a doubly good thing to work the body under lockdown restrictions as well as connect to people from other parts of the world. Since we are now suffering a global pandemic, we can gain from this global world by learning new techniques of self-care and artistic crafts.

Gratitude Is the Heaviest Debt

Monday, March 30

ON MARCH 27, THE GOVERNMENT ANNOUNCED THAT THE TWO grand Hindu epics, the *Ramayana* and the *Mahabharata*, would be rebroadcast on Doordarshan. It was probably the first time in India's post-independence history that a government made such an announcement. The *Ramayana* was written by the sage Valmiki, around the fifth century, and the *Mahabharata*, the longest epic poem ever, was written by the sage Vyasa in fourth-century BCE. Both were written in Classical Sanskrit (as opposed to Vedic Sanskrit, used in writing the oldest Sanskrit religious texts, the *Vedas*). The *Ramayana* is the story of the exile-and-return of the prince of Ayodhya, Rama. Before his return he defeated the demon king, Ravana, who had abducted his wife, Sita. The *Mahabharata* depicted the war of Kurukshetra, fought between cousin brothers for the throne of Hastinapur.

Both these period dramas, broadcast in the late 1980s, had dated production values. The *Mahabharata* was slightly better, and more interesting as a political epic. I was not interested in watching any of it. But with so much talk around the broadcast, including jokes on social media, I succumbed. I usually sat down to work straight away with my morning cup of tea, but this morning I chose to begin the day with a random episode of the *Mahabharata* on YouTube. It was the sixty-sixth episode and it turned out to be quite illuminating.

The episode begins with an interesting conversation between Krishna and Karna, against the backdrop of war looming over the kingdom of Hastinapur. Krishna raises the question of dharma/a-dharma (righteousness/unrighteousness), reminding Karna that he has always abided by the laws of dharma, while Duryodhana does not. Karna clarifies that his relationship with Duryodhana is not based on the question of dharma, but friendly affection. After he is humiliated by being called a charioteer's son (lower in the caste hierarchy), Duryodhana alone stands up for him. It is an act of claiming that Karna feels indebted to. Krishna acknowledges that gratitude is the heaviest debt but asks, is it a good idea to repay that debt by ignoring the question of truth and dharma? Karna says, he should have thought on that question before accepting the debt.

Karna's sense of debt is premised on a friendship that challenges his humiliation. Since the humiliation is based on caste, it has a wider social and political resonance. Karna is indebted to a friendship that treated him as equal among men (or, among upper caste, Kshatriya warriors). Duryodhana acknowledged Karna's skill and ignored his caste identity. Karna was indebted to that gesture. Krishna brings up the question of dharma. But he does not question the unrighteous act of the Kuru princess in declaring Karna unfit *by caste* to challenge Arjuna. Caste hierarchy is an accepted idea within Hindu dharma. The idea of equality is alien to it, and humiliation a norm. Karna suggests that he is indebted to Duryodhana's *act* and not necessarily his whole character. So, the question of Duryodhana's unrighteousness does not have a bearing on his debt.

In another scene, Kripacharya, Drona and Bheeshma discuss their unfortunate predicaments in the face of war. They are joined by Vidura, who declares that he is resigning from his post of Chief Counsellor (Maha Mantri). Bheeshma airs his frustration regarding his own inability (as the grandsire forced to side with the Kauravas) to resign as the grand commander of the Kaurava army. He laments that his oaths bind him to responsibilities. Vidura raises issues with Bheeshma's oath to protect the throne of Hastinapur. Bheeshma accepts the folly that while taking his oath to protect the throne, he hadn't anticipated having to protect (the interests of) a king like Dhritarashtra, whose blindness is a metaphor for his blindness toward the eldest of his sons, Duryodhana. Bheeshma's oath is typical of feudal times. Instead of pledging to safeguard the interests of the people, Bheeshma pledges allegiance to power.

Bheeshma's predicament reminds me of the Indian Constitution. Unlike in Bheeshma's time, the Constitution appoints the people as sovereign. But in a representative democracy, the government rules *in the name of* the people. If a government wants to tamper with the Constitution to suit its own ideology, it is entitled to do so. The Constitution can be restructured to suit power. In the hands of a man blinded by power, the law can be turned against the people.

THESE QUESTIONS OCCUPIED me till dinner. I stood for a while on the terrace after dinner, feeling the fresh wind brush against my face. The wind was a blessing. The delayed Delhi summer was a blessing too. It was still cool in the night. Despite the speculation that the Covid-19 virus may become less effective in high summer, it was difficult to wish for Delhi's cruel heat.

The street below was empty. Only a lone dog was lying in a corner. Before, when looking at the empty street late at night, you knew it would come to life in the morning. But now, irrespective of the light or the darkness, the sun or the moon, 10am or 10pm, the street had the same, empty look. The lone dog looked sullen. Even dogs must be wondering why the streets are empty all the time. A man appeared on his balcony, bored and lost under the light. Suddenly a whiff of smoke trickled out from below. My neighbour was smoking. She had enough cigarettes now to last her for a few days. Smoking is an act of existential meditation. We spoil our lungs, inhaling life's angsts. Our body must pay for the way we bear life. Life is difficult business.

How long shall we have to bear the lockdown? Will it be extended after twenty-one days?

Questions without answers are full of worry. I was calmed, remembering the tweet by Sara Jefry:[68] 'Your grandparents were called to war. You're being called to sit on your couch. You can do this.'

In these times, the best inspiration comes from what brings a smile to your face.

Of Masks, Montaigne, Alcohol & Friendship

Tuesday, March 31

TODAY I PROPOSED AN IDEA TO TWO FRIENDS ON WHATSAPP: LET'S have tea together in the evening on Zoom. They were game for it.

Suddenly it was 5.30pm, the appointed time for our meeting. It was too late for me to make tea. After a few moments of trying to figure out how to use the app (all of us using it for the first time), we settled down.

Mohinder Singh, who taught politics in JNU, was having his Darjeeling tea. Jitendra Kumar, a journalist and translator, and his wife, Bijoya, who works in public health, were sipping their own. Jitendra is also a good cook. He excels in cooking chicken (with curd) for large gathering of friends he invites, especially during the festival of colours, Holi.

We reminded ourselves of the pictures Mohinder had sent us, of almost empty roads in JNU, taken on his phone while taking a walk in the evening. He had sent them with a caption: 'When the air quality in Delhi is the best in decades, everyone is wearing masks.'

The mask has brought new and ironic complications since the arrival of the pandemic. France, a country receding into racism, had banned the hijab and the niqab in 2010. The mask has been declared mandatory in public spaces from May 11, 2020. However, the ban on the burqa, niqab and other religious forms of face and head covering will stay. The mask is justified for health or medical reasons. Masks have become identifiable with life (or protecting and saving life). But the burqa and niqab is dismissed as religious belief and practice. It is acceptable to cover the face for a bio-political reason (where life is put under the administrative power and control of the government) — as if the burqa and the niqab symbolize not life as such, but a form of culture that is expendable. The majoritarian argument is that cultural life is not crucial to the idea of life. Biological life, bereft of cultural marks is acceptable for public order. Someone may argue that the idea of religion in a secular society belongs, strictly speaking, to the private sphere.

Even by that classical definition of secularism, the tyranny of the French argument deliberately limits the meaning of "private" regarding the cultural rights of Muslim women in public in spatial terms. The private is not just the home. The private is any space where the individual owns the right to be herself. Private right includes who you are, and choose to be, in public. A secular society is not secular if it disallows cultural difference in public life. France is playing a dubious game with the idea of secularism.

There are other interesting aspects the arrival of the mask introduces to public culture and social interaction across the world. It requires a little history.

The journey of the mask as a performative object since antiquity to its modern, metaphorical existence is a fascinating one.[69] In classical Roman theatre, "mask" was understood as "persona", a word that came from Latin. Classical theatre was closed down during the sixth century by Emperor Justinian.

The reasons were ecclesiastical: Theatre was seen by the church as a corrupting influence of the Devil. When it reopened, the conceptual meaning of mask was no longer derived from the Latin "persona" but the Arabic, "mashara." If persona meant play, the mask represented a more deceptive quality. When theatre moved through the Middle Ages into the Renaissance, the mask went through its own transition from real object to metaphor. The mask was finally able to graft itself onto the face.

In the modern spectacle on stage, the face became the mask. It became the metaphor of identity. The masked persona chose to or was forced to veil the truth of the person. She also became the figure of guile. Every face was a mask, and every mask a face. To find the truth of a person meant "unmasking" him.

It reminds me of Ingmar Bergman's 1966 film, *Persona*. The principal characters, Elisabet, an actress, and Alma, a nurse, are heavily masked by interpreters of the film (including a famous one by Susan Sontag). Let me add a suggestive note to the story: Elisabet is under the vow of silence. Her vow is her persona. Alma (in Latin, meaning to nourish, nurture, foster) bares her soul (and her secrets) to Elisabet. Her persona bears her words/speech. Since the meaning of "persona" is closer to play than deception, the two women portray the two sides of language: speech and silence. The idea that personas hide something (else) beneath them is a shallow problem of objectivity. Personas may hide layers that you keep peeling to discover nothing. Each layer of our persona is as real and true as the subsequent one.

Yuko Mishima wrote the autobiographical *Confessions of a Mask* in his twenties, which earned him international fame. It is about a timid boy in Japan growing up to face his homosexual feelings in World War II. In Mishima's case it was a writer unmasking himself through his writing.

According to Nietzsche, the opposite is true. In *Beyond Good and Evil*, he writes: 'Every philosophy also conceals a philosophy; every opinion is also a hiding place; every word is also a mask.'[70] Behind every confession of the truth lies another façade. The face is also a façade.

The post-lockdown world of masks along with social distancing will be paradoxical. Eyes are the windows to trust. But eyes that you trust (or distrust) are part of a face. You trust the whole face of the person. If the face is masked, the eyes are masked too. There is a range of poetic literature on the eroticism of the veil. There are also Muslim feminists disowning the veil as a sign of property, the denial of sexuality, and objectification. The medical or health mask is not erotic, but utilitarian. It obstructs the sensuous visibility of someone's face. Even if a face is a façade, it is an open façade. A mask will close it to the world. A mask worn in public will turn people into aliens and intensify alienation. The irony of our times: It is now necessary (even compulsory) to mask yourself, to be an alien to keep yourself and others safe.

IN THE AFTERNOON, I received a message from Amandeep. He wished to share important information with alcohol lovers feeling deprived due to the lockdown. He sent a traditional recipe of this homemade beverage: 'Take two tender coconuts, strain the water and collect in a jar. Add five teaspoons of sugar, half teaspoon yeast, and stir well. Cover with cloth and fasten with a rubber band. Leave it for twenty-four hours. Voila!'

I passed it on to interested friends as my alcohol diet for the last few years has been restricted to white wine. They thanked Amandeep with effusive words of gratitude. Alcohol lovers don't lie, and they mean their exaggerations.[71]

THE LOCKDOWN IS a tale of many ironies. Mohinder was happy to suddenly find all the time in the world to read. Classes were suspended. Online classes were not possible, as most students did not have Wi-Fi.

Jitendra spoke of the article he was writing. In the context of how police humiliated citizens on the road after the lockdown was declared, he quoted Ram Manohar Lohia, the socialist leader who took part in the anticolonial movement. To paraphrase Jitendra: Lohia said, the elite in India followed the ruler's diktat by making it appear as an adjustment while the poor would follow orders anyway. Power in India was not concerned with how it treated people.

The conversation had an unexpected addition. A friend, Himanshu Pandya, who teaches Hindi in a mofussil town in Rajasthan, joined the chat. He was a bit distracted, however. The wine shops were closed, and the professor had run out of stock. His craving was further provoked when Mohinder informed him he had got enough to last him for a while. During our meeting, however, Himanshu managed to arrange something with a contact of his. We knew he had got lucky from the beaming smile on his face. Even his thick, short moustache beamed with anticipation. Thick moustaches are associated with either authoritarian men or satirists. The former wields more power. But satirists like Himanshu will have the last laugh.

The episode that unfolded before my eyes reminded me of nights in the university. We would frequently run out of alcohol. In the middle of the night, summer or winter, we would ride our bikes to the locality of a bootlegger. He would sell ordinary whisky or rum in quarter bottles at twice the rate. We took enough to salvage the party till dawn.

Excusing himself, Himanshu took his leave. I told him he didn't have to feel guilty. Even the great Urdu and Persian poet, Mirza Ghalib, was clear in his head that God will arrange for food, but we alone will have to arrange for alcohol. It was a matter of human responsibility.

Friends and alcohol make a trippy combination. But the association doesn't always last long. I think of the friendships I lost along the way. In school I would think all genuine friendships, like all genuine loves, were forever. I don't remember if I understood genuineness as something that exists in the heart, something you can feel, or that had depth. When I started writing poetry in high school, I would write only love poems and I would use the word "eternity" a lot. The idea of eternity ended with college. Neither love nor friendship turned out to be eternal.

It took time (and alcohol) to realise that not all friendships acquire fullness. Not all friendships measure up to a full bottle of alcohol. You also have half-friendships, half-loves, quarter-friendships, and quarter-loves. Friendships and loves are intoxications. Some last longer than others.

Comparing friendship to love, the popular French Renaissance figure Michel de Montaigne writes, love is 'more active, more scorching, and more intense', but also 'an impetuous and fickle flame, undulating and variable'.[72] Love, Montaigne writes, is limited by the fact that it seeks 'a fleshly end, subject to satiety'.[73] In contrast, friendship is 'general and universal warmth, moderate and even... with nothing bitter and stinging about it'.[74] The fever of love is considered absent in friendship. Friendship runs by tempered emotions. Perhaps the crucial difference lies in what Montaigne — quoting from Cicero — makes between love and friendship: 'Love is the attempt to form a friendship inspired by beauty.'[75]

The world has not come to grips with beauty. We desire beauty, but are prone to lose sight of it. Beauty has remained difficult to bear or set free, and hard to savour. Friendships, however, are hardly ever stable. I have seen them sway precariously in the winds of time. Friendships in our society are not exempt from 'the icy water of egotistical calculation',[76] a fiercely metaphorical expression used by Marx and Fredrich Engels in their famous political treatise of 1848. Friendships either strike a fine balance, or crack if they lack honesty.

In *Living to Tell the Tale*, García Márquez wrote about his friends with playful candour: 'Alfonso was viewed as an orthodox liberal, Germán as a reluctant free-thinker, Álvaro as an arbitrary anarchist, and I as an unbelieving communist and potential suicide. But ... even in the most extreme circumstances we might lose our patience but never our sense of humor.'[77]

Friendships based on strict ideological proximity suffer from sameness. Márquez and his friends did not suffer from this puritan idea of friendly comfort. Disagreements not only help you grow, they are fun. In JNU a lot of activists ("comrades" belonging to different shades of the left) herded together on party lines. Friendships between people who came from the same region and shared the same mother tongue tended to be boring. Friendship based on cultural, regional, or class familiarity is limiting. The moment you leave home, you look for the unfamiliar. You seek those who are a bit unlike you.

Friendship is a cuisine made up of contrasting elements. Someone with an aromatic personality is clove. Someone intense is cardamom. Someone delicately sensuous is cinnamon. Someone readily available, turmeric. Someone mild but edgy, nutmeg. Someone refreshing, coriander.

In the last few years, since the coming of the Hindu right, friendships have come under strain for political reasons. I don't judge a friend by his morality. It concerns them, not me. But a political belief that is harmful for others, and treats others as enemies, is a serious ethical problem. One should consider a person a friend or lover, irrespective of what the world thinks of them. It permits "too much world" between yourselves. You must judge a person, *alone*. The herd that puts people on trial is a beast without ears. Judgement is a matter of individual conscience and taste. There must be a measure of exclusivity in love and friendship.

Hindi movies have a lot of sentimental stories (and songs) based on friendship. Often these friendships get embroiled in bitter rivalries. Despite the exaggerations, these instances have a sobering effect on young people. Popular culture offers us glimpses of both the unattainable and the avoidable. Between the two, we mimic the emotions of friendship — imbued with motifs of masculinity and sacrifice — between Jai and Veeru in *Sholay*, Sher Khan and Vijay Khanna in *Zanjeer*, among others in the popular imagination, and we sing along.

The Cruellest Month & Food as Aphrodisiac

Wednesday, April 1

THE DAY BEGAN QUIETLY AND REMAINED QUIET. I KEPT WRITING at my desk, occasionally looking out of the window. The sky was bright and there was a breeze. After a while, I went on the terrace. A company of parrots was sitting in a tree. They would occasionally burst out like a fountain in all directions, and then return to their branches.

Covid-19 has posed a danger to human life. Watching ourselves, we are also watching other forms of life. In a way, we are reconnecting with our place in a world that is not just ours. We are reconnecting to a time when we had eyes and ears for others. The arrogance and indulgence that comes with power has blinded humans. Fear of illness, which, in a sense is to already live in illness, to be ill in dreadful anticipation, has opened our eyes. Mortality is a fact of life. But human beings are not used to living in biological fear. In this hour of discomfort, nature provides us with clues. The clues are simple, but decades of indifference have made it difficult to read them. Habit constrains the body, as much as the mind. It is time, says the virus, to open our eyes to nature.

T.S. Eliot's poetic reminders on time in *East Coker*, its patterns and imagistic moments, are inspired (or stolen) from *Ecclesiastes 3*. We know from *Ecclesiastes 3: 1–8*, there is a time for everything, but especially, 'a time to embrace and a time to refrain from embracing.'[78] The time to refrain from embracing is our time of the pandemic, the hour of physical distancing. In *East Coker*, Eliot presages this:

> Our only health is the disease
> If we obey the dying nurse
> Whose constant care is not to please
> But to remind of our, and Adam's curse,
> And that, to be restored, our sickness must grow worse.
>
> The whole earth is our hospital.[79]

The image of a nurse who is dying as she cares for a patient evokes the disturbing image of a pandemic. The curse of expanding sickness does not echo an individual crisis but a collective one. Covid-19 has reduced the world to hospitals and quarantine zones. Eliot's dark poem, published in 1940, was written during the war. His period of collective despair and death easily translates into other dark times.

We enter April, what Eliot called the 'cruellest month' in his long poem, *The Waste Land*. First published in London and then New York in 1922, the shadow of World War I falls on the poem. The poem's famous beginning, declaring April to be the cruellest month, was an upturning of the opening lines of the prologue to Chaucer's *Canterbury Tales*.[80] Chaucer welcomes April after the natural drought of March. Eliot, with his wife, Vivien, had caught the flu during the second wave of the same flu epidemic of 1918 that devastated Nirala and affected on Woolf.

The Waste Land, we learn from Elizabeth Outka, Professor of English and author of *Viral Modernism: The Influenza Pandemic and Interwar Literature*, is not just a poem about a land ravaged by war, but also by a pandemic. Her new book on pandemic literature reads Eliot's poem as delirium-literature, as a 'fever dream',[81] a corpse's tale. Images of death pervade the poem. Our April is perhaps also the cruellest in more than a century: Death, lockdown, thousands of migrant workers walking miles on hungry bellies, a nationwide virus of anti-Muslim sentiment, even health workers in danger of being infected by coronavirus and assaulted in the streets, a growing mental health crisis, and more. We have limped backwards toward Eliot's poem.

I RETURNED TO the topic of birds with my friend Bidhan, a teacher of political science in a college in Delhi. He was returning my call, not having picked up an hour earlier. I asked him how he was doing. He mentioned the sudden influx of birds around the kitchen garden in his small courtyard. Note, I asked how *he* was doing, and he talked about birds. I am reminded of Emily Dickinson:

'Hope' is the thing with feathers —
That perches in the soul.[82]

Birds, birds, everywhere, but not a soul in sight. Yet, my friend is happy with his soul, with birds around him. Satyajit Ray's film, *Kanchenjunga* (1962), also comes to mind. I had first seen it at the Sunday afternoon screening of regional films in Doordarshan during high school. There is a character in the film, Jagadish Chatterjee, who carries with him a book on birds. He is trying to locate a rare bird by its call. The film is set in Darjeeling, a place in the hills of north Bengal considered a retreat for Bengalis living in the city. Bengalis were the first community to mimic the British sahibs who made them the babus of colonial rule.

There is also the poem by Mahmoud Darwish, where we encounter the limits imposed on ourselves, but not on nature:

Here the birds' journey ends, our journey, the journey of words, and after us there will be a horizon for the new birds.[83]

After us, there will be nature, as nature is. The language of our presence has disturbed the natural balance of things. We lost our own balance.

I COOKED "PABDA" for lunch (the scientific name being Ompok Pabda). It's a fish of delicate taste. I shallow-fried it and used Peyajkoli in the curry. When I cook fish, I always add slices of ginger separately, later (not along with garlic in the beginning). I learnt this from my mother. Fried garlic tastes best in fish and meat. But since fish has a lighter taste, it is better to have the ginger (sliced or coarsely ground) thrown into the gravy so that it smells fresh.

The lockdown has affirmed that the most important thing I have discovered in life, besides reading, is cooking. I have been finicky about food ever since childhood. It took an hour to persuade me to gulp down my morning milk. The old man from Dhaka who worked in my railway colony home in Assam, Naresh da, was patient, and had enough stories to distract me whenever I was being fussy about milk or dinner. He did not have enough stories to last through my demanding childhood, so made clever variations, and often had no tale at all. He would begin slowly, deliberating on the telling of the story until my last morsel, and then stop abruptly. I would protest, but it was too late. I was a curious child and Naresh da intrigued me. I would watch him light up the clay stove and cook. Once he told my mother, "You don't have to worry about him. He will learn how to cook."

My inspiration to cook came from watching friends in JNU. I watched Bidhan and his Meitei friends cook pork during our evenings in the company of India's special contribution to the world of dark rum, Old Monk. The peeling of garlic and ginger, the cutting of onions and tomatoes, the smell of bamboo shoot and fermented fish, produced aromas fit for the gods. But the lazy gods won't cook for themselves. Good cooks are worthier than gods. I must have made mental notes watching them cook. Later, I met people at JNU who were cooks with distinct styles.

Jaishankar, from Kerala, did not believe in using the spoon to pour the masala. He measured the amount with his eyes. He made excellent spicy chicken curry. He would fry the chicken in a pan after roasting the masala. In another pan, he would fry sliced onion with ginger-garlic paste in mustard seeds and pour in the roasted chicken.

I asked him once, "What makes a good cook?"

He replied like a Zen Master. "One who knows the right amount of salt."

Mohinder, patient and thorough, was particularly good with

mutton korma and chicken biriyani. He preferred the Delhi style biriyani. He confessed that at one point he wouldn't attempt to make biriyani if one of the ingredients was unavailable: black cumin, black cardamom, green cardamom, mace, peppercorn, cinnamon, saffron, bay leaf, cassia, curd, mint. He has relaxed that stringent rule, somewhat, and now makes do with whatever ingredients are available in the kitchen. It is good to be flexible.

Zaheer is a food connoisseur. I have seen him cook dry meat with a stirrer in each hand during high summer.

When I started cooking, I discovered the second most important thing in human culture, after sex. Both cooking and sex have similar demands: a sense of aroma, patience, timing, passion, and a sense of balance. Writing shares these aesthetic virtues, literally and metaphorically. Patience, the nose for a good story, blended with the right ingredients, and stirred to perfection on paper, makes cooking akin to the art of writing.

The theme of food as aphrodisiac is explored by the Mexican novelist Laura Esquivel in her novel, *Like Water for Chocolates*. Fifteen-year-old Tita de la Garza pines for her lover, Pedro, who lives next door. Pedro asks for her hand in marriage. But the proposal is rejected because of a peculiar family tradition. Instead, Pedro is invited to marry Tita's sister, Rosaura. Pedro agrees, because it is his only chance to be near his love. Tita, who was born in the kitchen, loves to cook. Erotic love and passionate cooking get fiercely entangled in the household.

JNU HAD A film club that often organised screenings of avant-garde films. I remember once attending a screening of Sergei

Eisenstein's *Battleship Potemkin* (1926), but quickly realised I was not in the mood for it. I stepped out for a cigarette and waited for a friend still watching the film. I was relieved when the film finally ended and people were coming out. I overheard a conversation: A senior student, later to become a professor, was telling someone he had already seen the film several times. "But I came for the commitment," he said, raising his fist.

What was clear to me was that the commitment was not to cinema, but ideology. Eisenstein was the symbol of Russian communism in cinema and it was for this reason the patron troubled himself to watch the film again. I felt pity for him. Commitment is an empty gesture, one that in this instance entailed showing his face at a film screening as if attending a political rally. He had not come to the film to deepen his understanding but to be part of the grand dream.

I have a fondness for Jean-Luc Godard's *Breathless* (1960), notably because of actress Jean Seberg. She is casual and intense, airy and revealing. Perhaps the most endearing thing about her character is that she openly lives out her contradictions.

I watched a short interview with Seberg dated July 2, 1960, for the French television programme, *Cinépanorama*. The interviewer was curious about Seberg's recent visit to a private clinic. Seberg was candid as to why she was at a clinic for a week, but the interviewer was keen to make the actress confess to being psychoanalyzed. The interviewer's presumption, made in a public broadcast, was evidently wrong to Seberg, a sensationalizing of mental health. The Federal Bureau of Investigation took active interest in damaging Seberg's public reputation because of her political support for the Black Panther Party. The modern state executes more ruthless means than the church to endanger a woman's psychological and moral status if she does not toe the line. Seberg's association with a left-wing black movement alarmed the FBI. A woman celebrity in democratic America is not allowed to make political choices that may irk some white American men.

I realised, watching *Breathless*, that I was aware of Jean Seberg some twenty-four years ago. During my masters in JNU, I had visited Fact & Fiction, a bookstore that no longer exists. I picked up a copy of Carlos Fuentes' autobiographical novel, *Diana*, for no other reason than the image on the cover intrigued me. Diana Soren, the heroine of the book, was a mercurial Hollywood actress whom Fuentes compared to Diana, the goddess of hunting in Roman mythology. Leaving aside the many aspects of the novel, Diana is an invention based on Jean Seberg, with whom Fuentes had a brief affair during her shooting of a bad Hollywood film in 1970, *Macho Callahan*. One of the unusual details of Diana's sexual persona is using what Fuentes calls "fruit creams" as a sexual fetish:

'I would discover strawberry, pineapple, orange flavors, reminding me of the ice creams I loved to lick, when I was a boy, in a marvelous ice cream parlor... She made marvelous use of this bizarre commercial product, fruit-flavored vaginal cream which my imagination could take hold of.'[84]

The idea and image of the body as a fruit-flavoured platter melts in the imagination. In the world of commerce, the idea of (and demand for) aphrodisiacs undergoes a further artifice, becoming a marketing product. Desiring bodies can't escape slipping into the charms of commodity fetishism.

Light the Candles

Thursday, April 2

SINCE THIS MORNING, THE COUNTRY HAS BEEN ANTICIPATING THE prime minister's next speech, to be delivered at 8pm. He was being satirised on social media as the 8pm Prime Minister.

Yet another article appeared in the media on the Spanish Flu of 1918. It is estimated to have killed between seventeen million and eighteen million people in India alone. The Hindi poet and writer, Nirala, was twenty-two-years-old when the pandemic hit. In his memoir, *A Life Misspent* (originally published in 1939, the English translation appearing in 2016), he recounts the nightmare: 'The Ganga was swollen with dead bodies. At my in-laws' house, I learnt that my wife had passed away.'[85] In two striking lines, Nirala gives us an impression of how a deeply personal loss is a mere drop in the ocean. Pandemics turn death into something biological. *Who* dies is dissolved into *how many*.

Further, Nirala writes, 'My family disappeared in the blink of an eye. All our sharecroppers and labourers died, the four who worked for my cousin, as well as the two who worked for me. My cousin's eldest son was fifteen years old, my young daughter a year old. In whichever direction I turned, I saw darkness.'[86] Not just family, a life-sustaining world disappeared before his eyes. Such largescale deaths make grief bewildering.

THERE ARE ALSO episodes described by Gandhi that relate to the plague that hit India in the late nineteenth century. In *An Autobiography or the Story of My Experiments with Truth*, he mentions the plague of 1894 that broke out in Bombay (now Mumbai) raised concerns in Rajkot, where he lived. Visiting a Dalit locality in Rajkot to inspect their toilets, Gandhi was 'delighted'[87] to see they were kept clean. In contrast, the toilets in upper-class quarters, and a Vaishnava *Haveli*, were filthy. Clearly, the upper castes living by strict rules of cleanliness and needed others to clean their toilets, were callously negligent about hygiene. Gandhi reports on what he saw in the Dalit quarters: 'The entrances were well swept, the floors were beautifully smeared with cow dung, and the few pots and pans were clean and shining. There was no fear of an outbreak in those quarters.'[88] Cow dung, besides being used as fuel, is considered a disinfectant in Indian homes.

Gandhi also mentions how a ship in which he was travelling, the *SS Naderi*, was quarantined in port in Durban in December 1897. The authorities took precautions as the plague had reached Bombay before the ship left its shores. Part of the reason for the quarantine was to encourage the ship to return to India. Entertainment was arranged for the stranded passengers. On Christmas day, the captain treated everyone to dinner. After dinner, Gandhi chose to speak on western civilisation, and confessed: 'I knew that this was not an occasion for a serious speech. But mine could not be otherwise.'[89]

8PM. ALL THAT the prime minister had to say to the nation was to light lamps and candles at 9pm on Sunday, and keep non-essential lights turned off for nine minutes. This was met with immediate speculation, and jokes about the numerical significance of the nines.

As I am not dictated by rationalism, I don't mind what the scientific world calls superstition. Gabriel García Márquez was once asked about a statement he had made, that if one doesn't believe in God, one must at least be superstitious.[90] Márquez reiterated why it was a serious matter for him: 'I believe that superstitions, or what are commonly called such, correspond to natural forces which rational thinking, like that of the West, has rejected.'[91] Despite being a fierce communist Márquez stuck to his cultural roots, and proved his credentials as a writer who was aware of his anticolonial sensibility.

But the triumph of rationality over superstition does not account for an easy break within western history. In 1665, the bubonic plague hit various parts of the world, including London. In March 1722, Daniel Defoe published his defining account of the pandemic, *A Journal of the Plague Year*. Although widely acknowledged as historical fiction by scholars, the observations in the book merit our attention as they are part of the historical and cultural perspective of an English trader, writer and journalist in the seventeenth century. The narrator (and witness), H.F., is a saddler who trades with merchants dealing with the English colonies in America. Early in the book, H.F. describes how a terror-ridden people facing the avalanche of the plague is exploited by 'Fortune Tellers, Cunning Men and Astrologers, to know their Fortune, or as 'tis vulgarly express'd, to have their Fortunes told them... and this Folly, presently made the Town swarm with a wicked Generation of Pretenders to Magic, to the *Black Art, as they call'd it*'.[92] Despite being a religious man, H.F. calls these practices 'blind, absurd and ridiculous Stuff' and 'Oracles of the Devil'.[93]

Defoe's condemnation of supernatural practices echoes — and can be traced to — John Calvin and the Reformation in the middle of the sixteenth century. Weber defines the reformist influence of Calvinism in terms of the 'rationalization of the world, the elimination of magic'.[94] It clearly influenced the sensibility of seventeenth-century England.

Despite the tricky ways of fortune tellers and astrologers, who benefited from the fears of the populace, we can't miss the point that in a time of crisis, people looked for mental solace and signs of hope that could not be defined by rational considerations. In such a decisive moment, people in seventeenth-century England yielded to what Márquez calls the 'natural forces' of superstition.

Left-wing writers and intellectuals in India lack the confidence of Latin Americans like Márquez. They take pride in the (borrowed) idea of western rationalism as a yardstick of progressivism. This alienates them from their own culture. The idea of culture can't be a straight road inhabited solely by preachers of rationalism. The road must also have soothsayers and magicians. To quote Márquez again: 'I'm a timid writer. My true vocation is that of a magician, but I became so clumsy while trying to do a trick that I have had to find refuge for my solitude in literature.'[95]

The statement, even as hyperbole, is instructive. As a writer, Márquez identified himself with the skills of a magician. His literature is closer to magic than reason.

To return to the prime minister's speech. He believes that

a few minutes of a minor spectacle — people lighting lamps on their balconies — will work as a cathartic release for people under lockdown, and is a smart way to stay connected to the people.

The real problem with the prime minister's choice of communication lies in its monophonic tone and language. He's decided he will only stick to the non-essential part of the lockdown and the pandemic crisis and leave everyone else to deal with the essentials. That is a strange decision for a leader. He does not have to give us statistics, but he can share the concrete steps his government is taking. Hope is not just a symbolic act. Hope lies in how a nation responds to a crisis. Even though there is nothing infantile in the act of lighting lamps and candles, it can suggest an infantile relationship between power and the people. The people are not children, delighting in light, sound and action.

RICHA AND I took a walk after dinner. It was our first walk during the lockdown. My friend, Bidhan, was right about the moon yesterday: "I have only seen the pale yellow moon in Delhi. The moon is finally silver."

Even though it wasn't a full moon in all its glory, the silvery glow was unmissable. Even the stars looked brighter, and nearer. It made the night feel more night. The street was also empty. I would have loved to walk a long way for a long time, but it was too late to venture far. I didn't want to be adventurous. We kept to our own street. Mother had called up twice during the week to tell me I must walk every day. I wasn't sticking to her advice, so I had mixed feelings of guilt and responsibility as I took the walk.

Cooking and washing dishes kept my hands busy. It was time

to exercise my legs. Writing for long hours takes a toll on the body. Keeping this journal has helped me to stay calm through the days but has also rooted me to the chair and the table. I haven't yet graduated to a laptop. I use my PC. I find the laptop keyboard too slippery. I will have to move to the laptop one day soon, but till then shall remain with the PC. I like its solidity and the pressure of the keys beneath my fingers. I also like the sound of the keyboard on a PC. It reminds me of the typewriter. The laptop keyboard is noiseless, like swimming. But I will wait for my day to swim.

Death, Famine & Morality in Satyajit Ray's Films

Friday, April 3

I REALISED HOW MUCH WRITING HAD HELPED ME TO ESCAPE THE boredom of lockdown. Cooking does not last for more than an hour and there are otherwise still empty hours to fill. Writing has helped float the boat. Friends texted me about their growing restlessness. Some, living in gated communities, couldn't even take a walk within the grounds. The paranoia of safety is such a paradox; it has no limits of its own but is obsessed about limiting.

I refused to have Netflix, despite the temptation. Netflix is a machine that encourages total occupation. It will eat into my writing time and paralyze me. I prefer to enjoy films in my own time, at my own pace. When my mind is working, I like to attend to it and read or write. I want to watch films when I feel free from myself. Film demands total attention, and I want to be ready for it.

A few years ago, I devoted a week to the films of Satyajit Ray. These were films of Ray's I had never watched or could barely remember. I saw them one day at a time: *Mahanagar/The Big City* (1963), *Pratidwandi/The Adversary* (1970), *Seemabaddha/Company Limited* (1971), *Aranyer Din Ratri/Days and Nights in the Forest* (1970), *Kapurush/The Coward* (1985), *Ashani Sanket/Distant Thunder* (1973) and *Ghare Baire/The Home and the World* (1985). After a sharp and memorable look at village life in *Pather Panchali/Song of the Little Road* (1995), Ray turned his gaze on the city. I won't forget my excitement and surprise while reading Saul Bellow's novel, *Herzog*, during my graduation days in Assam, where Bellow suddenly mentions Ray. I got the book from the well-kept library in the Audit department of N.F. Railway headquarters, where my father worked as a stenographer.

The central protagonist in *Herzog* is Moses E. Herzog, who undergoes a Nietzschean bout of misogyny and Dionysian frenzy, after his second divorce. Among other things, Herzog's state of madness leads him to write frantic letters to people alive and dead, to philosophers like Nietzsche, and even to God. The letters are often cynical and acerbic in tone. In one of the letters to an Indian, Dr. Bhave, Herzog writes: 'Recently, I saw *Pather Panchali* ... Two things affected me greatly — the old crone scooping the mush with her fingers and later going into the weeds to die; and the death of the young girl in the rain.'[96]

Herzog was watching the film in a New York theatre on a rainy day. Those three scenes are among others you associate with the film of striking imagery. Ray had the finesse to make scenes unsentimentally tender. Death has a face in *Pather Panchali*. But it is also a social condition. For the poor in the village, life's resources aren't enough, and death is always round the corner.

After *Pather Panchali*, Ray became a dedicated chronicler of middle-class (and upper caste) Bengali life. His films have cinematographic nuance. Some of his characters are well drawn. But he never reached the epic scope of his first film. His well-crafted films falter on a deeper issue: his preoccupation with middle-class morality. Ray's depiction of bourgeois realism is constricted by his frequent relapse into bourgeois idealism. Ray uses his women characters to mark and restore the film's idealist, or moral, contours. For instance, Madhabi Mukherjee in *Mahanagar/The Big City* plays a lower middle-class housewife, Aroti, trying to make ends meet. She has the added burden of an insecure husband and a prejudiced boss. The onus is on her to prove that her heroic individuality (sacrificing her job to uphold a value), matches her trustworthy wifehood. Sharmila Tagore plays the idealistic sister-in-law, Tutli, in *Seemabaddha/Company Limited*. When she learns that her brother-in-law, whom she respects and admires, was instrumental in endangering the lives of factory workers, she quietly returns the watch he had given to her. This symbolic note (moral and personal) is all that Ray offers by way of a comment on class hierarchy. Swatilekha Sengupta plays the housewife, Bimala, in *Ghare Baire/The Home and the World*. She becomes emotionally and sexually entangled with her husband's old friend, a fiery and seemingly idealistic political activist involved in the Swadeshi Movement. Realising that her husband, a mild mannered zamindar, is genuine and humane and that his friend, for all his fake machoism, is opportunistic and timid, Bimala draws herself back. Once again, the filmmaker uses a woman's sexual and (eventual) moral agency to comment on the dangers of a political movement. The psychological aspects of human life that Ray is so good with blunts under this form of cinematic resolution. Even though all three films are taken from stories written by others, Ray had enough creative licence to offer his own view. Bengali women had surely come a long way since Tagore wrote *Ghare Baire* in 1916.

I share these thoughts with Richa during dinner. She nods thoughtfully and comes up with an interpretation that would have impressed Susan Sontag: 'Ray is the women in his films. He can't empower them politically. So he meekly resolves the crisis in the story by using them as instruments of his moral sense alone.'

In the shadow of the pandemic, I am also reminded of Ray's film, *Ashani Sanket* (*Distant Thunder*), on the Churchill-orchestrated Bengal Famine of 1943 that took five million lives.[97] It is based on Bibhutibhushan Bandyopadhyay's story. Before the famine sets in, there is an episode where a man comes to meet Gangacharan, the Brahmin priest-physician-teacher rolled into one, for his help regarding an epidemic that has erupted outside his village, Kamdebpur, some nine kilometres away. Gangacharan conducts the rituals and warns the villagers not to drink from the river, and to throw away stale and rotten food. The Japanese invasion of Burma has a ripple effect on food supply in India, monitored by British control. It creates massive food shortages and starvation in the village. The mill owners and grocers hoard rice and refuse to sell any. The priest dissuades his wife from hand-pounding rice with other women to maintain caste distinction. Social status and prejudice must be preserved even at the risk of impending hunger.

The film's lens is upper caste, and the moral conflicts in the film stay within a caste sensibility.[98] When the Untouchable (Dalit) girl dies in the end, we experience her death through the hesitations of the Brahmin priest, Gangacharan.

The character Chutki is an exception to Ray's frequent relapse into moral closures. Chutki survived an earlier epidemic and gives in to the sexual advances of a scar-faced man, to acquire some rice. She discovers he was disfigured in a fire and tells him, "*Tor o dekhchi sohoje maron neyi*" (You too, I see, won't die an easy death). It is a stunning moment — disturbing and moving — that tries to evoke a kindred sense of fate, stitching the wounds of emotional and moral despair.

YET ANOTHER TRAGIC piece of news arrives this evening: A twenty-two-year-old student, Balasubramani Logesh, from western Tamil Nadu, died in Hyderabad last night, after travelling 450 kilometres over three days from Wardha, Maharashtra, on foot and other modes of transport. His death will remain among the reports, and he will be missed by his family and friends. Since the lockdown has been declared a necessary part of the "war" against Covid-19, any death caused by this war will be "collateral damage".

"Trust Begets Trust"

Saturday, April 4

Normally the Tablighi Jamaat passes each year without notice. This year the event is the hub of some controversy. The Tablighi Jamaat sees orthodox Islamic preachers coverge at the Nizamuddin Dargah but because of Covid-19 restrictions, and the presence of foreign nationals from hotspot countries, like Malaysia and Indonesia, it is believed the event has facilitated the spread of positive cases. Nearly one third of the spike in Covid-19 cases since the end of March are attributed to the Jamaat event. Authorities are trying to track down each attendee and quarantine them. It will be even tougher to identify each person's travel history and fellow travellers who might be infected. Social media did not waste time in demonizing Muslims. Hashtags like #CoronaJihad and #TablighiJamatVirus quickly circulated on Twitter. The virus was the perfect conduit to merge paranoia with the pandemic. Why would people endanger their own lives and the lives of others? The Jamaat can be accused of stupidity but not conspiracy.

Religious followers live in another era, often refusing to accept advice or listen to commonsense. For believers, Covid-19 may well be divine punishment. But then, one expects people to observe certain norms when it comes to possible danger to life. Any religious congregation is untimely and risky at such an hour.

You can't question or ridicule faith with a sense of superiority, however. Faith is not responsible for all the problems in the world. Often what appears to be a collective act of faith can be devoid of an inner spiritual quest. The spiritual is something personal, never collective. Faith is belief that offers meaning to life. It has both personal and collective dimensions. Religion includes discipline and the observance of traditional practices. These traditions are part of cultural habit. Religion also manifests in political structures. It becomes a code for subservience to certain political and social rules. Religion in this form is an ideology of power.

In the modern world, religion and political power often sit side by side. Colonialism, for instance, was/is a modern structure of power, in which religion is not essential. Colonialism is crudely based on exploitation for the sake of economic profit. There is nothing religious about it, though it can aid the propagation of a certain religion. Religion helps in the consolidation of state power. Theocracies are often run by corrupt men who rule in the name of a god. The modern era has shown us the blurry lines between what naïve, secular modernists consider as the rift between reason and religion.

With terrific accuracy and precision, the Romanian philosopher, E.M. Cioran, writes in *A Short History of Decay*: 'We kill only in the name of a god or of his counterfeits: the excesses provoked by the goddess Reason, by the concept of nation, class, or race are akin to those of the Inquisition or of the Reformation.'[99]

In a single sentence, Cioran brings the medieval and modern worlds of power to the same table. The names have changed, but intention hasn't. The secular world is as much a matter of belief as a religious one. It is tempting to quote Cioran again: 'A human being possessed by a belief and not eager to pass it on to others is a phenomenon alien to earth, where your mania for salvation makes life unbreathable.'[100]

This sentence is as true of religious missionaries as it is of virulent nationalists and communist ideologues. God has appeared in history as a torment, whether as an idea, a belief, or a metaphor. A party manifesto can be a holy writ for its followers. The stupidities that religious people are prone to may not be of the same kind as the stupidities of rational unbelievers. There are divergences in the way one understands the world. But look beneath the outward appearance of difference, and you will find the secret pleasures of collective brotherhood, an instinct for power, the arrogance of illumination — divine or rational. In such a world, prejudice comes from every side. The mad preachers of the modern world have sorted one thing for themselves: the refusal to acknowledge and learn from others.

PANDEMICS REQUIRE A pragmatism often missing in people of faith or in those who can be fatalists regarding the meaning of life. This can be seen in Defoe's *Journal of the Plague Year*. In the book, H.F. had decided to stay on in London, rather than move to the countryside, where people were retreating to escape the infection. H.F. had a business to look after with a shop and warehouse of his own, including a host of servants who were at his disposal. He read certain occurrences as signs from God to not undertake the journey, and placed his hope in divine providence to save him from the plague. His elder brother, a merchant just returned from travels in the Middle East and Asia, scoffed at his reasoning:

the Turks and Mahometans in Asia and in other Places... profess'd predestinating Notions and every Man's End being predetermin'd... (and how) they would go unconcern'd into infected Places and converse with infected Persons, by which Means they died at the Rate of Ten or Fifteen thousand a Week, whereas the Europeans or Christian Merchants, who kept themselves retired and reserv'd, generally escap'd the Contagion.[101]

Despite being a religious man, H.F.'s brother prefers prudence over fatalism. Since the time of Calvinism, debates on human (free) will had emerged in Christian society.[102] These debates and changing notions were likely to impact social life and lead to a secularity of beliefs. They also fostered the ethic of mercantile capitalism.

The representation of Turkish and Muslim fatalism by H.F.'s brother is aired with the confidence of an English trader. But this ironically does not prevent H.F. from belief in divine favour. During an evening of intense dilemma, H.F. submits to the verses of Psalm 91 in the Bible, which he interprets as God's reassurance: 'There shall no evil befal thee, neither shall any plague come nigh thy dwelling.'[103] There is, however, a tacit material attachment to his business in London that underlies H.F.'s succumbing to a fatalist impulse derived from doctrinal authority.

It is difficult to draw conclusions about collective behaviour based on faith. There needs to be a deeper historical and social understanding behind the complex behavioural patterns during a pandemic; why some are more alert than others during a time of such crisis. Every religious society professes doctrines of predestination, yet their psychic responses to the pandemic may be materially determined.

Interestingly, in situations that provoke collective fear, the idea of free will that marks the shift from a religious to a modern, secularised society, is understood in negative (or passive, self-preserving) terms: as self-restraint, a will of reasoning against exposing oneself to danger.

IN INDIA, THE behaviour of the Jamaat was seen through a paranoid and accusatory lens. Even Hindu groups congregate over religious rituals. Religious groups are prone to congregational habits. They live by it. Faced by a pandemic, such groups can look to religion for solace and solution. Congregations cannot, however, jeopardize public safety.

People belonging to religious communities, who live by congregational culture, may find it difficult to suddenly give up their practices even in the face of a medical emergency. It creates a corresponding spiritual emergency.

The individualist nature of the modern world finds it easier to cope with the demands of social distancing, unlike traditional societies. The point is not to dismiss the nature and necessity of congregations out of modern, individualist arrogance.

DISTURBING REPORTS POURED in from different parts of the country that health care workers were assaulted, and even spat on.[104]

There is social stigma, collective paranoia and ignorance

behind such acts directed at people who risk their lives to take care of others. The disgust is pathological. Fear becomes instigation and an excuse to mistreat others.

There is also mistrust of any intrusion of social or private space. This mistrust is often political in nature when it involves poorer sections of the minority community that live with a sense of threat. If a political establishment does not instil trust in its minorities, we cannot expect the feeling of trust to be reciprocated. As Gandhi wrote in his weekly English journal, *Young India*, on June 4, 1925, 'I believe in trusting. Trust begets trust. Suspicion is fetid and only stinks.'[105] If the air is infested with hate and distrust, frontline workers are likely to bear the brunt. There is no justification for any collective behaviour that borders on violence. It is our social responsibility, as much as the government's political responsibility that people breathe the air of trust. Or else, even in a pandemic crisis faced by everyone, the fetid air of suspicion will corrode people's hearts.

Chernobyl, Bhopal & the Gospel of Reason

Sunday, April 5

9PM. THE PEOPLE WHO PRIDE THEMSELVES ON REASON AND deride the prime minister's call for lighting lamps as mere superstition, are curious and alert on social media when the allocated time arrives. The intelligentsia uphold a sense of hope that is amusing: that any criticism will be heard, valued, and considered. Politics needs innovation, but social media prevents it from rising above easy rhetoric.

The intensity on Twitter was palpable. There is nothing wrong or ugly about lighting candles and lamps; there is everything wrong and stupid about firecrackers. My neighbourhood responded calmly. At 9pm some households switched off the lights in their living rooms but in other houses you could see lights. People in one building were evidently not keeping track of time. They were late in switching off their lights. Apart from one flat on the second floor that had enough lamps to light up their balcony, most houses only had one or two candles. Clearly no one had ordered extra lamps or candles for the occasion. The moment the allotted nine minutes was over, one young man chanted from his balcony, "*Bharat Mata Ki Jai*" (Victory to Mother India). The sentiment was echoed from the balcony of another building nearby. There were not more than two or three voices, followed by firecrackers. An event supposed to restore quiet hope and poignancy, had turned bizarre. Social media was filled with an outpouring of celebration and derision.

I was disturbed but could not help feeling amused. People were bored and frustrated. They were desperately trying to feel upbeat. An untimely sense of jubilation was overtaken by a false sense of bravura. Maybe people did feel powerless. People felt trapped in little cages. The world had turned into a zoo, with one notable difference: no visitors were allowed in. Covid-19 had upset the prevalent mood of hyper-nationalism in India by introducing a strange, unexpected biological time that threw everyone into the same ring of fire.

LATE IN THE night, I decided to watch my first film under lockdown: Werner Herzog's documentary, *Meeting Gorbachev* (2018). I skipped dinner to finish the film. Herzog followed the life of the former Russian President: his peasant upbringing, his father a war veteran. Gorbachev talks about the occupation and destruction of Stavropol by the Germans during the war. Wheat was difficult to grow, and the first postwar harvest was poor. The famine of 1946–47 made it worse. Gorbachev's great early achievement was the successful opening of the Stavropol canal in 1974, which even Stalin had failed to achieve. It brought him to the notice of the politburo and Brezhnev in Moscow.

The explosion of the nuclear reactor at Chernobyl in April 1986 was Gorbachev's moment of truth. The city of Chernobyl is situated twenty-five kilometres north of Kiev, in Ukraine. The hazardous radiation emanating from the explosion led to the evacuation of around 30,000 people in Pryp'yat and, over time, caused thousands of cases of radiation-induced illness. Scientists estimated that the zone around the plant wouldn't be habitable for 20,000 years.[106]

Gorbachev took the devastation more seriously than politics. Or rather, his understanding of politics was shaped by the devastation. Gorbachev acknowledged the calamity of Chernobyl as "one that we cannot forget". That was a great admission by a leader. In India, leaders preside over human disasters, including engineered riots, and forget all too easily. The fate of a great nation and a petty one depends on the capacity of its leaders to face the truth.

A disaster like Chernobyl influenced a humane leader like Gorbachev. It also produced a great writer in Svetlana Alexievich. Alexievich produced an oral history of those who had experienced Chernobyl, speaking of how they had lost their town and their lives. Imagine a place where death was a daily topic of discussion. It was not just a question mark on the Soviet Union's scientific projects, but on science itself. In the last section of *Chernobyl Prayer*, Svetlana allows the narratives of children to merge in a nameless choir. The language falters between innocence and pure bewilderment. It is a difficult read. One child wonders if God has punished her because she did not tell her mother that her "new dress got caught on the fence and torn".[107] Another child tells us: "The first year after the accident... sparrows disappeared. They were lying all over the place, in gardens, on the tarmac. They got raked up and taken away in containers, along with the leaves."[108] And, "My best friend was called Andrey. He had two operations, and then they sent him home. He was supposed to have a third operation in six months' time. He hanged himself with his belt, in an empty classroom... 'We will die and become part of science,' Andrey used to say. 'We will die and everyone will forget us.'"[109]

The disappearance of life and habitat, a dread of becoming the object of scientific enquiry — of *becoming science* — and being forever cast from memory, underscores the boy's fears. It is a horror of people becoming alien. Science must be more responsible to life.

THERE ARE UNCANNY similarities between what happened in Chernobyl and Andrei Tarkovsky's Soviet science fiction movie *Stalker* (1979), made seven years before the disaster. The main disaster site of Chernobyl was officially called The Exclusion Zone. The cordoned-off, hauntingly empty and forbidden area in *Stalker* is referred to as the Zone. The mysterious site full of abandoned objects, overgrown vegetation and stagnant water seems to indicate the aftermath of a disaster. The heavily guarded entrance to the Zone suggests it is a state secret.

In the film, the protagonist, a writer, tells a woman he meets that the world is "ruled by cast-iron laws [and] insufferably boring". He says the Middle Ages was interesting, with its churches. "Because if God is also a triangle," he says with a truly epic sense of humour, "then I don't know what to think." The writer alludes to the fact that people were suddenly faced with a new form of abstraction in modernity (and Russians, more specifically, under the communist regime), where symbols of religious faith were replaced by scientific language as a new form of belief. The writer finds this idea of God, as a measure of truth taken over by a quantifiable idea of mathematical figures, as absurd.

In his essay on Fyodor Dostoevsky, Octavio Paz wrote that communist ideologues in their rejection of Dostoevsky were 'intent on making society a square and each man a triangle'.[110] The God of the modern era is a (scientific) formula. The church has been replaced by a much more businesslike and toxic place: the laboratory.

In any civilisation that goes by the principle of "trial and error", disasters like Chernobyl or Bhopal are bound to happen.

If Chernobyl found its writer, Bhopal found its poet. In his book of poems, *The Whiteness of Bone*, Jayanta Mahapatra reflects on the Bhopal Gas Tragedy of December 1984, where thousands died because of toxic gas leaking from a pesticide plant. In 'A Morning Walk in Bhopal', Mahapatra writes:

> A road, going somewhere
> cranking silence from the morning light
> or perhaps from the autumn of my fear.
> At times I see someone walking down it
> looking at me through the skies of my pain.
> That road leads to the edge of the earth
> where water slips with sad voice and falls...
>
> Now with what longings
> shall I protect my memory?
> whose presence
> keeps moving with my breath?[111]

Mahapatra paints a wreckage of time. The desolate landscape disturbs him. It offers a sadness that turns into amorphous images, weakening the poem. But you can still hear the clarity of water that 'slips with a sad voice and falls'.

In 'Bhopal Dawn', the poet writes about the body: 'Tapped inside, Dreams / build still, tense into the light / which leads to unimaginable damage.'[112]

It is a dawn shrouded by death. In the poem 'The Hill', Mahapatra draws the unforgettable image of how 'with hundred-year faces / the orphans of Bhopal stare at the lost hill'.[113] Faces of stone, transfixed by the effects of radiation, age lifelessly. The gaze is fixed on the site of painful wonder. What went wrong?

In 'Death of a Nameless Girl in Bhopal, December 1984', Mahapatra writes:

There has always been starvation here, man;
yes, we are used to it. This pain was new, one
of the loose ends. And obviously
sanity seems necessary.[114]

It is possible and necessary to read the poems against the effect of scientific disasters. Science has no memory. Memory has no science. Science is an idea of progress without memory. Memory is a shelter. Memory looks for shelter. When a scientific experiment goes wrong, it affects nature. The sky, the sunlight, and even the silence, turn toxic. The effect on human body and life from an industrial-scientific project gone wrong can be as damaging as war. People live in a daze and the body becomes alien. The 'new' pain with 'loose ends' that Mahapatra describes can only be understood as a miscalculation that occurred in the laboratory of 'progress'. Those who swear by the gospel of science will blame mismanagement for the problem. But a clearer view can't ignore the dangers of science.

THE GOSPEL OF Matthew in the New Testament reads: 'Jesus answered, "It is written: Man shall not live on bread alone, but on every word that comes from the mouth of God."' (Matthew 4:4). The poor do not live on bread alone, either. They live on the tyranny of words that come from the mouths of the masters (be it employer, police, etc.). The world must be rid of surrogate gods. God does not speak, but listens. A book is holy because it was written. What is holy is language. If we earn our bread, we have earned the right to words. The bread we have brought to our table and the words we have learnt to speak count in equal measure. We don't need the help of rationalists to understand that. We need faith in ourselves, and each other. Reason has merely twisted the gospel to its advantage: 'Man shall not live on faith alone, but on every word that comes from Reason.'

But science and reason hasn't ended exploitation, hunger, hatred or racial prejudice. It has brought us war and other scientific disasters. We need to be cured of the gospel of reason.

In *Devils* (also translated as *Demons* and *The Possessed*), Fyodor Dostoevsky gives us an invaluable critique of reason through the artful technique of using one character speaking for another. Though Dostoevsky has also aired his views on the subject in other works, including *Notes from Underground*, he makes the definitive point in this novel. In an excited conversation, Ivan Pavlovich Shatov, a believer who struggles to be faithful, cuts down to size Nikolay Vsyevolodovitch Stavrogin, whom Shatov once admired as his political idol, but who turned out to be someone who had "lost the distinction between evil and good".[115] Summing up Stavrogin's thoughts, Shatov says:

'Reason has never had the power to define good and evil, or even to distinguish between good and evil, even approximately; on the contrary, it has always mixed them up in a disgraceful and pitiful way; science has even given the solution by the fist. This is particularly characteristic of the half-truths of science, the most terrible scourge of humanity, unknown till this century, and worse than plague, famine, or war.'[116]

What Dostoevsky says about the moral ambiguity of reason is reminiscent of Hannah Arendt's brilliant insight about fascism that 'most evil is done by people who never made up their mind to be either bad or good'.[117]

The charge against reason by Dostoevsky is a startling one, because with reason we can define and distinguish things. But Dostoevsky thinks that clarity has eluded rational thinking when it comes to ethical matters. Rational arguments on right and wrong action are too neatly drawn and don't offer ethical directions for the heart and mind of an integrated human being.

John Stuart Mill in his essay, *On Liberty*, proposes his 'harm principle', and writes, 'the only purpose for which power can be rightfully exercised over any member of a civilised community, against his will, is to prevent harm to others.'[118] Such a statement conveniently ignores historical (and ethical) crimes like colonialism and racism. Mill's 'others', instead of the victims of colonialism and racism, can very well be those who rule over them.

In the eventful history of the long twentieth century, the meaning of human life has disappeared into the black hole of reason.

Memory, History & the Tunnel of Schoolmates

Monday, April 6

I WOKE UP LATE. THE LAST TWO NIGHTS I SLEPT LONGER THAN usual. I felt drowsy throughout the day. Waking up late is detrimental to any sort of activity, including writing. The days are passing in a daze anyway. One is adjusting to life, and one's relationship with the world. Earlier, when we texted friends or spoke with them, we learnt how life on the end of the line was different from ours. Now, everyone has been forced into a common situation. Life is indoors. We face the same difficulties and concerns for the future.

The state of inertia enables recollection. I thought of the conversation I had sometime in March. I had allowed myself to forget it the moment it was over. It had interrupted my day the moment it had begun. I wanted to put it in safekeeping and leave it for another time. It came out of the casket today. Conversations with people you once knew deeply may weigh heavy in the memory. You reflect on them later, as time eases the weight. Memory often returns suddenly, like a bird that perches on the electricity wire. We have a secret place for storing memory and summon it at will.

A cow re-chews or re-swallows food, what we call chewing the cud. Human beings chew the cud of memory. It is also called rumination, and memory is part of the mental activity of rumination. Chewing cud improves the cow's digestion. Ruminating on things, including things past, allows us to draw useful lessons in the present.

LISTENING TO CHOPIN'S *Nocturnes* during lockdown enables a gentle flow of recollections. I am amazed by what these twenty-one pieces for solo piano do for memory. Each time I play *Nocturnes*, some street, or face, or moment, or mood belonging to the past, gently trembles in my head.

Music brings back memories. But Chopin's *Nocturnes* does it at a subtler level. The music does not overwhelm you. It reconnects you to the past the way a hand holds yours and persuades you to travel along. Listening to Chopin, I could "hear" the distinction between emotions and feelings. Emotions stir the blood. Feelings correspond to what surrounds you and introduces a greater ambience. Feelings connect you to the air, to nature. You can almost observe yourself, if not exactly in the objective sense. You observe with the sensuous attachment of one watching an intriguing film. Unlike emotions, feelings leave you with a space to wonder. As does the night.

I GOT UP late, my mind vaguely awake, as I remembered the call I had received from an unknown number. I picked up the phone to the booming voice of a man who initially refused to name himself. He asked me if I recognised his voice. I did but ignored the question. There were other voices behind his and I soon realised this was a party line. The voices belonged to old classmates from school. I deliberately hadn't kept in touch with them. I had met some of them a few years back and we did not have much to talk about then. We were only connected in memory and past time. I loved those days at school, still do, and feel awful to have outgrown them. I love the way one falls in love in school, tormented by so many hesitations. Those hesitations are our first lessons of love. Friendships never followed any rule. We made fun of each other, like siblings. When rules are relaxed, life is easy, yet we are sensitive. Too many rules spoil the broth of life.

I did not want to stay in touch with classmates from school because I did not share anything of value with them anymore. I did not share the same jokes. And I did not share their present idea of the world. I heard, with a pang of sadness, how some of my classmates had abandoned their secular adolescence. I did not want to spoil my nostalgia.

It was predictable, because once you grow older and settle down to middle-class luxuries, you can afford a thick skin. It is time to abandon the idealism of your formative years.

Everyone thinks they can graduate in history by reading blogs run by charlatans. The internet helps the wide circulation of trash by individuals and collective propaganda machines. The most disturbing aspect is that people feel empowered by excitable versions of history that foster hate.

I remember conversing with an old friend and senior schoolmate via email, around 2012. After personal titbits on life and romance, we strayed into discussing politics. He sent me certain blogs with ungrounded facts and wild exaggerations to acquaint myself with Indian history. When I told him I didn't need these as I had spent nine years in the JNU library reading history books, he told me those history books were full of lies. I was shocked by the effortless ignorance of his audacity. I had come across propaganda during childhood without knowing it was propaganda. My father was close to people who worked for organisations associated with the Hindu right. His uncharitable views on Gandhi and Nehru did not impress me. I equated his abrasive tone with ignorance. I preferred to listen to my social studies teacher and took her more seriously than my father. Years later, at JNU, I was exposed to pro-Chinese and anti-Tibetan propaganda, by left-wing ideologues. They had a "progressive" pretention to them, like all left-wing propaganda. Everything the Chinese government did was acceptable in the name of communism. Since Tibet is under the spiritual influence of the Lamas, their society is considered backward. But does that justify Chinese occupation of Tibet?

WHAT I HADN'T anticipated was the degeneration of public culture after 2014. Muslims were suddenly being demonised in filthy language in the public sphere. Even some of my Hindu schoolfriends, who grew up on Ghalib and Sahir Ludhianvi during our secular adolescence, aired Hindu nationalist sentiments. Poetry and the language of love were clearly not enough for political belief. A rich and complex history of India's encounter with Muslims was reduced to the bones of war. There was no longer a place for Amir Khusro's contribution to Indian music, or *Sirr-e-Akbari*, Dara Shikoh's bid to reconcile the monistic elements of Hinduism with Islam in his Persian translation the *Upanishads*, or Akbar's *Din-i Ilahi* ('Divine Faith' in Persian), a unique attempt made by a ruler in the late sixteenth century to create an ethic of (social) life from different religious traditions.[119]

Tagore was among the world's most remarkable critics of nationalism.[120] He thought the nation saps the 'living bonds of society' and serves a 'mechanical organization'.[121] The impersonal and alienating nature of the nation resembled, for Tagore, 'a scientific product made in the political laboratory'.[122] The nation is also a product of reason where a new experiment will be made to forge an abstract community loosely based on history. He contrasted this discomforting idea with a sensuous, medieval encounter between Hindus and Muslims:

> We had known the hordes of Moghals and Pathans who invaded India... as human races, with their own religions and customs... we had never known them as a nation... we fought for them and against them, talked with them in a language which was theirs as well as our own.[123]

Tagore's observation is borne out by history. Despite strife and bloodshed, mutual admiration and engagement contributed to the spirit of Indo-Islamic culture. The flagbearers of Hindu nationalism today want to deny the deep history of this cultural spirit. They want to build, decorate and run a new train of history. Erase the old track and construct a new one. They want to invent a new idea of paradise. As with most human constructs, paradise is an exclusionary idea: *You* have no place in *my* paradise.

The classmate on the phone asked if I recognised the other voices on the line. I said I did but gave no names. He named them himself. Everyone was speaking over the top of one another, their words breaking into bits and pieces. The logic of such a polyphonic conversation does not lie in the coherence of language. People simply adore the sound of nostalgia and familiarity. Half the call was spent on everyone shouting out each other's names. That was precisely the purpose: to recount the names of old days. Some voices dropped off the line and couldn't reconnect. I was alone with the original caller again. I told him, "Since the doors of the present are currently locked, you felt like opening the doors of the past, eh?" He laughed, "Exactly."

He had told his wife about the time he stayed over at my hostel room in JNU for a night and our lunch at the library canteen the next day. I asked how he felt about the current situation in the country. He said things were happening in the right spirit. I asked him about the most current problem: the plight of workers stranded between city and home. He acknowledged the problem, but said with conviction that there were enough buses to take the migrants home and that many families, including his own, who lived near the bus stop where workers had gathered, were offering them food. Every problem is solved by the morality of the good citizen. I probed deeper and asked what about the minorities feeling insecure in the country. He acknowledged that "a few wrong things" had happened but stated that the responsibility of a good citizen was to convince people of the greater good for the sake of the nation. For him, Covid-19 was an opportune moment of nationalist revivalism. He had figured out his squares and triangles. Once the larger dream was accepted, everything else was a matter of mathematics.

Childhood is deceptively simple. Our ties with it become more deceptive as time goes on. As I recalled those voices on the phone, I visualised a tunnel, where faces were lined up, one behind the other. They were inviting me to join them. It was a tunnel of echoes and I did not want to enter it. I did not want to lose myself in the echo of voices, each imploring with a touch of paranoia and uncertainty, *hello? hello?* I had abandoned my childhood and did not want to revisit it.

The past is as hollow as the voices on the telephone. It would be hazardous to return to the classroom, or to the football field, or to the many roads and culverts of evenings spent together in youth. I want to encounter the past only in memory, not in the real world.

Of Moustaches, Forgotten Clothes & Sadness

Tuesday, April 7

I WOKE UP LATE AGAIN.

Mohinder had asked me to look at a short story by the Hindi writer, Agyeya (the non de plume of Sachchidananda Hirananda Vatsyayan). He said that the story, 'Daroga Ameechand,' written in 1938, provided "interesting clues to the nature of power". I looked online and found the story in Hindi.

The story is about a much feared tyrannical inspector of the Hazara jail, in Punjab, Ameechand. He had a commanding presence, accentuated by a handlebar moustache. He would test the sharpness of his moustache with a lemon. If the lemon was punctured the moustache was suitably sharp. One day pebbles are discovered in the daal at the prison, and the prisoners protest. They want Ameechand to investigate and refuse to follow rules until he does. Ameechand gives word that intimidatory tactics won't work and some prisoners are punished. But the rebellion continues for a month and news of it spreads. Ultimately the Inspector General decides he will pay a visit. Ameechand declares a truce with the prisoners. One old prisoner suggests they should take back their demands but make a new one: the Daroga must lower the edges of his moustache before them. Ameechand has no choice but comply. He meets with the prisoners and curls down his moustache. When the Inspector General visits the jail, the prisoners are rubbing their upper lips and guffawing. He remarks to Ameechand that his prisoners lack discipline, and the Daroga is transferred. But wherever he goes, the story of his deflated moustache arrives ahead of him. With his reputation in tatters, Ameechand takes early retirement.

Power draws strength from symbols. Once the symbol of Ameechand's power, his moustache, is diminished, his power is also diminished. The Daroga wasn't aware of the significance of his moustache and that tampering with it might affect his power. The daring of the old prisoner also played a role in unsettling the dynamic between the Daroga and the other prisoners. It weakened the Daroga psychologically. Ameechand's willingness to listen to their demands was circumstantial, fuelled by the Inspector General's visit. The prisoners ensured that the lowering of the moustache, like the lowering of a flag, contributed to Ameechand's symbolic defeat.

I shared my thoughts with Mohinder on the phone. He provided his own insight, saying that "power ultimately hangs on something very fragile!" Ameechand's moustache was notorious and formidable. But his ego was fragile. Ultimately, his moustache could not bear the weight of his bruised ego. Masculine power often lies in fragile symbols of pride.

Osip Mandelstam's poem, 'The Stalin Epigram' comes to mind. Written in 1933, Mandelstam describes Stalin in the language of folklore. The poem is so visibly derisive that it can make even children laugh. Yet it also evokes horror.

Among the lines in the poem is this one: 'the huge laughing

cockroaches on his top lip.'[124] It is probably the most unsettling image of a moustache in all literature. Stalin's ego must have been particularly hurt by the line because the poem cost Mandelstam his life. He had made it difficult for Stalin to live with his moustache. There is no doubt that Stalin took as much pride in his symbol of masculine power as the fictional Ameechand had. Mandelstam had lowered the status of Stalin's moustache, and his pride, before the world.

Satyajit Ray had once translated a poem written by his father, Sukumar Ray, the famous nonsense-rhymer. The poem was about a clerk who, on waking up one morning, declared that he had lost his moustache in his sleep. He refused to believe the mirrors his subordinate workers held before him, and trying to assure him to the contrary. The last three lines are a perfect (nonsensical) rationale to the delirium:

> What Man is to Moustachio:
> Man is slave, Moustache is master,
> Losing which Man meets disaster![125]

Moustachio is the official symbol of machismo.

THE DAY PASSED quietly as usual. There were occasional texts from friends who wanted to share a thought, or piece of news. I was mostly occupied in writing. In the evening, I took a fresh shirt from the wardrobe. Another everyday activity had disappeared: We have no reason to change our clothes as frequently as before. I hesitated a moment before I pulled the door of the wardrobe open, seized by a strange feeling. What if I find instead of clothes skeletons dangling from the hangers? I was amused by the thought. I felt almost embarrassed to meet my clothes. It was as if I had opened a closet to my past life. The clothes were familiar, but they never looked so remote before. There was a mix of summer and winter wear, both appeared alien. Summer clothes had never appeared so distant, not even in winter. I felt the fabric in my hand with the nostalgia of a man dreaming. I felt I was touching clothes I had worn in another life, as if I had forgotten they had ever existed.

THE AFTERNOON TRIGGERED memories, like a film that someone has suddenly switched on for you. I fell in love at school. Love was the discovery of joy and sadness at the same time. I was happy I was in love, and I was sad to be away from her. To exist separately after you fall in love is something no advice or knowledge can help you reconcile with. I thought all sad songs were written by people like me. I learnt to hum and remember those songs almost out of a sense of duty. I thought the singer Kishore Kumar knew me best. He was the ventriloquist of my sadness. It was a typical story of love in a small town.

I was also sad when parents or uncles and aunts scolded me at home, or teachers at school. I felt they berated me without knowing my heart. I felt misunderstood. I felt my friends alone understood me, but only sometimes. I realised there was no escape from being alone. That sadness grew over the years. It made communication difficult. I was always fumbling for words. For a while, I lived freely. Even though I spoke a lot in those years, I still could not say what I really wanted to say.

I used to stammer as a child. My tongue used to get caught, especially in vowels. Grown-ups teased me because of it. They made me stammer more without realising their own ignorance. Speech was difficult. It aided writing. Writing is often born out of the difficulty of speech. Talk wants more talk and more life, more endless evenings. But ultimately it falters and falls to its knees. I felt spent in speech and retired to writing. I became a shadow leaning over a notebook at a table, gathering words.

Years later I discovered Constantine Cavafy. His poem, 'Hidden Things,' was a revelation. I found solace in the opening lines:

> From all I did and all I said
> let no one try to find out who I was.
> An obstacle was there distorting
> the actions and the manner of my life.
> An obstacle was often there
> to stop me when I'd begin to speak.[126]

I used to wonder if Cavafy stammered like me. My obstacle in life was my shyness. I froze between my lines before a crowd of students, the only time I had reluctantly agreed to take part in a poetry recitation competition. I was even anxious during the taking of the attendance register. I hesitated to speak to girls, for fear of my tongue getting stuck midsentence. But my shyness was not natural. It was born of my hesitation, my fear of mockery. My shyness held my tongue. Cavafy's poem holds the key:

From my most unnoticed actions,

my most veiled writing—

from these alone will I be understood.[127]

There is hope, if not an altogether promising sort of hope. Cavafy accepts that loneliness can only be overcome in writing. If writing alone will deliver the language of my solitude, so be it.

Someone at university gave me a practical solution in the form of a simple mantra: I should pause a second before opening my mouth to speak. I learnt to steady my breath and became more confident.

Reading the poet K. Satchidanandan one day, I felt I had finally reached the heart of the matter. His poem, 'Stammer,' offers an important clue. 'Stammer is the silence that falls / between the word and its meaning.'[128] Yes, I know this silence. The poet then asks, 'Did stammer precede language / or succeed it?'[129] It is not a question concerning the origin of language, but the *act* of language. Perhaps our ancestors stammered into the first syllables that became the first language. Stammer as speech is a fascinating idea, one that disturbs the grammar of language. Satchidanandan writes, 'God too must have stammered / when He created man. /... That is why everything he utters/...stammers, / like poetry.'[130] Satchidanandan is telling us that it is impossible to express the language of emotion without any hesitation. Love is the stammering of language.

Since adolescence, I have loved to meet people for the sake of conversation. Young people, old people, friends, strangers, anyone I could listen and talk to. I listened as much as I spoke. I was keen to learn about others. I wanted to know their sadness. When you listen attentively to young people, they tell you what makes them sad. People believe those who listen. I learnt everyone has a different reason to be sad. We are prone to sadness and there is no lasting antidote. Conversations without ambition, without reason, are a curative.

The modern world aided the flowering of individuality on the stage of equality. We brought the differences of our identities and our lives, to the table. We heard and learnt from each other. We went back home desiring each other's company. We discovered difference, not just as points of conflict or repulsion, but also as a beautiful enabler of desire. We broke the barriers of identity and age. We laughed at the older world where everything deserved either suspicion or reverence. Our open, rebellious world grew paradoxically closer and further apart with technology. The internet introduced us to a shadowy world where people were free to lie to one another. Distrust bred a faceless medium of interaction. Strangers entered the privacy of the household and created new ways of escaping (and rebelling against) bourgeois conservatism. The internet also brought a new solitude, and the paranoia of technology.

Every era has a last station. Then the train moves backwards, its engine attached to the rear. Our sentences stop making sense. We are sentenced for our language. We were sentenced by our language. Words rolled backwards on our tongue. The era stammered.

I HAD GROWN my hair during lockdown. There was also a visible patch of grey beard. I could have shaved but I let it be. I thought of my hairdresser, Mazhar. We would always have a lively chat about politics whenever we met. He was quite vocal about his politics in the salon. The last time I met him was after the Delhi riots. He was terribly upset by how Muslims were facing persecution.

As Mazhar cut my hair, the shorn locks covered his arms or drifted to the floor. Hair can be so attractive on a person's head, but the moment it is cut away can appear revolting. It puts me in mind of a striking line by Osip Mandelstam in 'Ariosto': 'Power is disgusting like a barber's hand.'[131] Despite the arresting imagery, I feel Mandelstam uses the barber's hands unfairly as an image of disgust.

Mazhar reminded me of Akbar, the barber who first cut my hair, when I was a boy in Assam. Father would take me to the salon. Of the barbers there, I only wanted Akbar to cut my hair, no one else. A small stool was placed on the barber's chair on which I could sit. I would blabber constantly as Akbar worked on my hair. It was difficult for him to keep my head still. Everything was a distraction for me, including the radio playing Bollywood songs. I would hum along with a familiar song. The barbers enjoyed my childish propensities. A trip to the barber was never a chore or mundane. It was a richly evocative place and carnivalesque. There were jokes and opinions on everyone from celebrities to politicians.

We also shared a sense of persecution. Bengalis were called "foreigners" during the Assam Movement. We were refugees from erstwhile East Bengal. My father had migrated to the Indian side of Bengal after Partition. He came to Assam in 1951. As the earliest beneficiaries of the colonial administration, Bengalis found easy work on the railways. It was a point of resentment for the local community. Biharis were also considered "outsiders" in Assam. The eastern state of Bihar provides India with a large (and cheap) body of migrant labour. When I was growing up in Assam in the 1970s, we mostly had Bihari men as rickshaw pullers, barbers, gardeners and bearers. They were also sack-lifters in wholesale markets. I won't forget the humiliation of the Bihari banana seller whose basket was upturned in the street by local boys, just for fun.

The barbers were Muslims from Bihar. That was no reason for distance. We did not need to share a religion for a haircut. We spoke to each other in Hindustani, a mix of Hindi and Urdu. My father and Akbar would share common anxieties about the political situation, often with a touch of humour. A visit to the barber was an occasion for stories.

I resigned myself to the fact that I needed a haircut. The summer heat made it itchy, and the humidity did not help matters. I picked up the scissors and trimmed my hair carefully to achieve a crew cut. Trying my hand at being a barber, I realised more than ever why I need a barber. But I am not completely dissatisfied with my work. Just as I had learnt to cook by observation, I have been a keen student of the barber over the years, curiously following his deft moves with the scissors. I finally had a shave too and decided to finish off this ritual with a bath. Then I got back to my desk.

A SHORT ESSAY has been published today in the *Paris Review*, 'Sheltering in Place with Montaigne' (April 7, 2020), by Drew Bratcher, a writer and editor from Nashville. The subject of the piece is Michel de Montaigne, the great sixteenth-century French statesman and writer. Montaigne's *Essays*, published in 1580 in three volumes, is a landmark in European literature. It influenced a host of great writers across disciplines, from René Descartes, Blaise Pascal, Jean-Jacques Rousseau, and Friedrich Nietzsche to Virginia Woolf, and even Shakespeare.[132] Montaigne's central preoccupation in *Essays* is to offer an ethic for living, embracing human imperfectability. Bratcher states that Montaigne wrote his *Essays* under the shadow of plagues, political uprisings, the deaths of people close to him, and his own health issues. Bratcher calls *Essays*, '(part) evolving treatise, part prismatic self-portrait,' which for Montaigne 'was the antidote to self-isolation, a recurring conference in the midst of quarantine'.[133] Perhaps this is why, I thought, he sought brighter experiences. Why else would Montaigne write, 'I fear a stuffy atmosphere and avoid smoke like the plague'?[134]

Montaigne had a noteworthy predecessor. In the essay, 'Of Smells,' Montaigne informs us, 'We read of Socrates, that though he never left Athens during many recurrences of the plague which so many times tormented that city, he never alone found himself the worse for it.'[135]

The Absence of Absence

Wednesday, April 8

I FINALLY TOOK THE TIME TO PONDER THE INCREDIBLE GALLERY OF photographs on the lockdown, published by the *New York Times* on March 23, 2020, under the striking title, 'The Great Empty.'[136] Apart from the emptiness of space, in certain photographs, like the one by Andrew Testa of a street in London, and one by Laetitia Vancon on a subway in Munich, the claustrophobia of modern spaces is apparent. It is the claustrophobia of high buildings and enclosed concrete spaces. I wonder what it does to our senses in "normal" times. It is evident that such spaces rob us of natural light, and we spend time under artificial lights even during the day. Day is night. It must influence our wellbeing.

In a photograph by Gilles Sabriée, we see a young man dining alone in a Beijing restobar. I wonder what prompted him to visit the place: habit perhaps, or lack of food at home, boredom, lethargy or inability to cook. He looks intently at his food in the picture. It looked to me as if he were not simply alone in a bar, but alone in the world. The bar was the world. Philip Cheung's photograph of the empty beach in Santa Monica offers a metaphysical point of difference: A crowded beach belongs to the world. An empty beach belongs to the universe.

The photograph by Maria Contreras Coll of a pavement in Ras Ramblas, Barcelona, shows pigeons on empty roads. The pigeons look dull and disinterested, despite having the streets to themselves. Boats in Srinagar, photographed by Atul Loke, have sat empty since August 5, 2019. There is no trustworthy word from God or government. The boatman looks like he is waiting for an answer from the mountains. It is a long wait over land and water. The train standing in the Rawalpindi station, photographed by Saiyna Bashir, is as empty as the yellow bin on the platform.

In her book, *On Photography*, Susan Sontag writes: 'A photograph is both a pseudo-presence and a token of absence.'[137] But in the photographs I am describing, there is a double absence: the absence of the photograph superimposed over the absent reality (or absent presence) of human beings. The absence of absence. In the photographs that feature in the *New York Times* article, we see what is not there, yet which exists within the image regardless — anguish.

The last image that holds my attention: Two, probably three people seated in a near-empty theatre in São Paulo, photographed by Victor Moriyama. I always long for a similar scenario in Delhi, where people come to watch a film, but prefer to get busy with their phone, and constantly order food. They treat the theatre more like a restaurant.

I was lucky to find my wish fulfilled while watching the film *Photograph* (2019), at Saket, back in March last year. The director, Ritesh Batra, received attention after his previous film, *Lunchbox*, (2013) premiered at the Cannes Films Festival and won the Rail d'Or. There were no more than five people in the hall. Still I could not escape the reason why I wanted a near-empty theatre: A man, sitting alone, was talking on his phone. The presence of others did not matter to him. The world was his home.

If he was asked by someone later, "Which film did you see?" I imagine him replying, "Oh, it had the actor, Nawazuddin. The name of the film slips my mind. I was on the phone."

The man must be quite unhappy today, under lockdown. He can't visit a theatre, where he can chat to his heart's content on his phone.

I RETURNED TO reading Pessoa's *The Book of Disquiet* after lunch, sitting in the shade of the terrace. The afternoon breeze was mild despite the growing heat. Still, the eucalyptus had a cooling presence. I noticed how people had slowly stopped appearing on their balconies, even for a brief while. It could be the heat. It could also be a sense of resignation: There is not much hope in the clouds and birds are no longer a distraction.

The affluent middle-class prefers furniture to nature. They love to pile up things in the house the way they endlessly feed their appetite. Dead objects inspire a certain hedonism, which may be partly explained by the drabness of daily life. The emptiness of life is directly proportional to the accumulation of empty goods.

I am struck by an undated entry in Pessoa's notebook:

Isolation made me in its own image. The presence of another person — one person is all it takes — immediately slows down my thinking ... A simple invitation to supper from a friend produces in me an anguish difficult to put into words... 'My habits are those of solitude, not men.' I don't know if it was Rousseau or Senancour who said that, but it was some spirit belonging to the same species as me.[138]

Pessoa suggests a personality that cultivates an aesthetic isolation. Loneliness enriches language, and company diminishes it. Not perhaps company itself, but the burden of speech in company. Pessoa imagines his semi-heteronym, Bernardo Soares, as a character who prefers silence to speech, and hence loneliness to meetings. Only when a man looks at a blank page is he confronted with the temptation to create. The presence of another person is an interruption to that possibility and delight. Pessoa's invented writer has close resemblances to Kafka.

In his *Diaries*, Kafka writes in July 1913, 'I hate everything that does not relate to literature, conversations bore me (even when they relate to literature), to visit people bores me, the joys and sorrows of my relatives bore me to my soul. Conversation takes the importance, the seriousness, the truth, out of everything I think.'[139]

Kafka tells us what he discounts as being literature: everything that does not suffocate is not literature. The joys and sorrows of his relatives are too facile to deserve his attention. They do not match up to the intensity of life that Kafka carries in his head. Truth is serious business, and there is no truth outside literature. Kafka's idea of truth displaces the Platonic idea. Truth is not an idea, whether of goodness or beauty. Truth is literature, and literature is the articulation of how one suffers life, and the world. Kafka's ideal state is contemplation in solitude.

For a writer addicted to solitude, even cordiality can be

oppressive. André Gide writes on an ordinary day in early twentieth century: "This morning lunch with Gosse at the Crillon. More wearing than pleasurable. The conversation exhausts me. Gosse is exquisitely cordial... Ah! I should like to plunge into a deep bath of silence."[140] For Gide, solitude is cathartic.

For Kafka, even the (sexual) expectations of marital life cause unease. In August 1913, he notes in his diary, "In me, by myself, without human relationship, there are no visible lies. The limited circle is pure."[141] Kafka is not exactly saying that human relationship is a lie. But in relations, one is often compelled to lie, to hide the truth of one's inabilities to match the expectations of others. This predicament tears Kafka apart. Truth is to express oneself fully, without fear or trepidation. Kafka discovers literature is the only means to talk about himself.

The lockdown would have pleased Kafka, as it would Soares, both acute solitude seekers. They would have enjoyed the certainty of not having their profound thoughts disturbed by friendly invitations to lunch or some such.

What would have bothered Kafka is to be locked in with a sexual partner, unless of course he had a room of his own, a door that could be bolted, and time at his desk. It is difficult to accuse writers like Kafka of conventional selfishness because they do not ask much from the world. All they want is a corner in which to be able to disappear. Even a gaze that falls on them a certain way can be enough to put them into despair. They are not mad. They are victims of an unnerving clarity.

The curfew would have affected Soares and his fondness for strolling around the city. Soares was a *flâneur* and loved taking walks. Though he abhorred company, he enjoyed being the discreet observer taking notes on life around him and sharing his thoughts with the reader.

HERE I MUST end with an interesting episode concerning the European obsession of solitude. In August 2001 I just started my PhD at JNU. My good friend, Ramesh, was leaving for a university in the United States to pursue a doctoral degree. I was among a few other friends accompanying him to Indira Gandhi International Airport in Delhi to see him off. On the way, I thought of the wonderful times and many conversations that Ramesh and I had shared. I recollected some of the remarks he had made over the years. Once, I had come to him with a story of the heart. It was late at night and I wanted to sit in his room and tell him of my heartbreak. But the moment he realised the nature of my story he immediately said we must go outside. I said I wanted to avoid going out as I didn't want us to be disturbed by anyone we knew. But Ramesh was firm. On seeing the hesitation and discomfort on my face, he said:

"Matters of the heart must be talked about only in the marketplace."

The statement had a magical effect on my spirit, and immediately I felt a little better. I could have almost done without the conversation that followed.

On reaching the airport, which was teeming with people, we said goodbye to Ramesh and gave him a hug before he departed for the check-in counter.

Among our party was Mohinder's German friend, living in

India. "Why do so many people in India come to the airport to see off someone?" he asked. "It gets unnecessarily crowded."

With a flicker of a smile, Mohinder replied, "Don't you think it is nice that people aren't left alone? People here make an effort to show that they care about you."

The German friend nodded in agreement, and said gravely, "You are right. Europe will die of solitude."

Treatise for the Wanderer & the Colour of Waiting

Thursday, April 9

AFTER LUNCH, I CALL A FRIEND WHO LIVES ALONE IN KUMAON, IN the hills of Uttarakhand. Nirmal Swaroop is a researcher in psychology and linguistics. It is a world like our own but resembles another. The sense of familiarity I once experienced when talking with him is something lost in the pace and bustle of city life. There is a 'secret bond between slowness and memory',[142] writes Milan Kundera, in *Slowness*. Swaroop, too, is interested in reconnecting with lost elements of his past life, and perhaps this is what slows him down. But it is also a matter of his temperament.

He tells me the plum, pear, peach and apricot trees are now ripe with buds. It is spring, and the weather is pleasant. The Hindi word for spring, *basant*, is a beautiful one. Basant is the name of a season. But in Hindustani classical music, there are ragas based on seasons that include the Basant raga.

I share with Nirmal my recent reading of Agyeya's short story. It prompts him to recite a haiku on spring by Yosa Buson, a Japanese poet and painter translated by Agyeya. Nirmal is surprised, but happy, that he remembers it. The original haiku in Japanese was written in 1782. Agyeya's Hindi translation goes: '*Varsha mein vasant ki maine dekha chata ek, ek barsati saath jaate batiyate.*'

The English translation, by Robert Hass, reads: 'Spring rain: telling stories, a straw coat and umbrella walk past.'[143]

Nirmal tells me that he wants to reconnect with Hindi. His reading in the Hindi language was over at the age of eighteen, due to the demand for English in higher education. He wants to freely hold on to both options. Nirmal mentions Rahul Sankrityayan, the brilliant literary travel writer and scholar. Sankrityayan would use pure Hindi and a mix of Hindi and English, at will. In a slim book titled, *Ghummakar Shastra* (*Treatise for the Wanderer*),[144] Sankrityayan said, so Nirmal tells me: One who wants to travel can't live by Brahminical rules. You must be ready to eat anything.

A man of such rules is in many ways an absurd misfit in the world. He complains that the world doesn't fit into his rules.

Swaroop wants to leave behind a trust run by a voluntary group that would offer counsel on mental health. There are only three doctors in Haldwani, the largest city of the Kumaon region, to take care of around 40,000 inhabitants. In a world forced into self-isolation, one that doesn't look like it will abate any time soon, there will no doubt be a greater need to address mental health.

THERE IS A ban on travel under the lockdown. The infinite wait is a matter of unspeakable despair for lovers. It is impossible to articulate waiting, except that you are waiting for a person you know, and you are fond of. You wait for someone's presence to bring you closer to life. Love is a heliotropic desire. It moves us towards the light of another person.

I happen to know a young couple who have been forced apart. The woman is trapped in Almora, where she had travelled for a work assignment. The man, who is a film editor, pines for her in Delhi. One of the activities they enjoyed together was cooking. Now the man cooks with half a spirit, while the woman is confined to a guest house where there is not the luxury of cooking. The lockdown has dropped between them like a gate at a railway crossing. The train of days rolls by endlessly.

The time of waiting is unlike any other time. It is a time of strangeness, where the person one is waiting for undergoes a change. Will you find the same person when you meet again? Will you be the same when you meet again? Waiting often changes you, temporarily. You do not simply wait to meet the other person but what you were with that person, in their company. You wait to find out about yourself.[145]

The situation for this couple is more acute than the situation Roland Barthes describes in *Lover's Discourse*. In their case, no one is making the other wait. Something else is. And yet, they are not free from the fundamental anxiety that Barthes describes: 'I am waiting for an arrival, a return, a promised sign... Everything is solemn: I have no sense of *proportions*.'[146]

When one waits, the colour of waiting is splashed on the wall and other objects.

On Love: Razia Begum, Shakespeare, Kiarostami

Friday, April 10

RAZIA BEGUM, A TEACHER IN A GOVERNMENT SCHOOL FROM Telangana, drove her scooter over 1,400 kilometres to bring home her son. He had been stuck in another town since the twenty-one-day nationwide lockdown was imposed. Razia drove over empty roads, carrying enough food to last her journey. The police, for a change, cooperated with her, and offered good advice. She was also carrying a letter from the Assistant Commissioner of Police, Mr. Reddy. Mr. Reddy had told reporters, "I was moved by her love for her son."[147]

The crux of the story lies in the *decision* of the mother to fetch her son. Once she took that decision, all other acts and possibilities followed naturally. A decision is necessary in both love and war. There is a threshold of "normal" life that must be crossed — needs to be overcome — to jump into the state of love and war.

TO FALL IN love is to fall into a zone of conflict. Conflict is an inescapable condition of the world. Love brings a state of conflict at many levels. There is a conflict within oneself, for instance, of how to be and not to be, of what to say and not to say, of how to act and how not to act, of what to think and not to think. The conflict in love is a self-conflicted one, between hesitance and expression.

Love also throws us into the world. Conflict might arise with others, often within the family.

'In our world,' Octavio Paz writes in *The Labyrinth of Solitude*, 'love is an almost inaccessible experience. Everything is against it: morals, classes, laws, races and the very lovers themselves.'[148] To emphasise the point, Paz adds: 'To realise itself, love must violate the laws of our world.'[149]

In Shakespeare's murkiest love tragedy, *Othello*, in the backdrop of an impending conflict (the Turks may attack Cypress), Othello is accused by the Venetian Senator, Brabantio, of wooing her daughter, Desdemona, using wrongful means. Othello defends himself calmly, claiming:

> She loved me for the dangers I had passed,
> And I loved her that she did pity them.
> This only is the witchcraft I have used[150]

Othello displays considerable honesty in his admission that Desdemona pitied the dangers of war, and that she was attracted by the quality to face and undertake risks. When it was her turn to speak in defence of her love, Desdemona said:

> My noble father,
> I do perceive here a divided duty:
> To you I am bound for life and education;
> My life and education both do learn me
> How to respect you; you are the lord of duty;
> I am hitherto your daughter. But here's my

Husband:
And so much duty as my mother showed
To you, preferring you before her father,
So much I challenge that I may profess
Due to the Moor my lord.[151]

Although set in the late sixteenth century, the sensibility is remarkably modern. The patriarchal father is acknowledged for Desdemona's 'life and education', which makes her duty-bound to him. Yet, for a woman, the question of duty, or loyalty, is complicated the moment her lover turns up. In this conflict, Desdemona has her mother's example to follow. The threshold of a woman's freedom is marked by the relinquishment of filial loyalties for the sake of love. It is a matter of preference. For Desdemona to describe Othello as 'the Moor' is no accident. It is a deliberate affirmation of her betrothal to someone who is considered an outsider, a man of colour, the other of white Christian Europe.

Defeated in argument by her daughter and her lover, a desperate Brabantio tells Othello as the couple make their exit:

Look to her, Moor, if thou hast eyes to see:
She has deceived her father, and may thee.[152]

Brabantio does not understand that love is not defined by fate, but by the *decision* the lovers take to risk their lives for love. His racial suspicions of Othello (that he can successfully woo her daughter only through witchcraft), is extended to a moral suspicion of her daughter. There is a calculated reasoning behind Brabantio's desperate bid to raise Othello's suspicions about his own daughter. But the delusional logic is also telling. The patriarch can't bear to realise that his power has been rejected by a simple, honest, human act. Since those in power rule by deception, they imagine the world is run by deception alone. That is why it is difficult for power to understand love.

RAZIA BEGUM'S DECISION threw her into the conflict beyond her doorstep. The letter from the police commissioner ensured that she could sail through the strict and hostile barricades, through the state of emergency. It was her passport to reach her son. A mother's love for her children is never in doubt, but the police commissioner was still "moved" in this instance by the conditions surrounding it. It was a courageous decision for a woman to travel so far, risking so many potential problems.

Love is never at peace. Love is the most intimate when we, as lovers, enact the conflict between nature and culture. The difference between war and love is the willingness to be vulnerable in love and surrender.

I remember the unforgettable last scene of Kiarostami's film, *Through the Olive Trees* (1994). A desperate and persistent Hossein first walks alongside Tahereh, the girl he is wooing for marriage, trying to convince her of his sincerity. But Tahereh, walking ahead of him, does not respond. Hossein is not discouraged by the silence. He is hanging on to the hope lodged in his heart. When Tahereh leaves him behind, he runs like a madman to reach her through the lush olive trees. The camera pauses on a longshot. Hossein and Tahereh are reduced to specks in a vast sea of green.

This is when she turns to tell Hossein whether she will accept his hand in marriage — an answer that we, the observers, cannot hear. The answer is sacred, and so deserves privacy. But we see him sprint back. No lover will run with such spirit if dejected. Hossein has risked insignificance to win a world. Why does Tahereh make Hossein run after her for so long? To see how far he can go to persuade his own heart. It is a moment worth living and dying for.

I WATCHED MY second film during lockdown with Richa, which happened to be Kiarostami's final film, *24 Frames* (2017). It is a fascinating conversation between photography and cinema. *24 Frames* epitomises Kiarostami's urge to minimise storytelling by offering the audience open frames of imagination. By digitally reconstructing moments before and after each photograph in four-and-a-half-minute episodes, the filmmaker contrasts stillness with movement.

The film is Kiarostami's quiet, artistic statement on the Anthropocene, understood as a geological condition where human influence has caused a gross imbalance in the natural environment. Kiarostami invites us to reflect on the disappearance of nature. He shows how the deer, the seagull, the sparrow, and even the lion, are doing fine on earth, except when their lives are interrupted by human presence. The film has an eerie connection to our pandemic condition. We are witnessing and experiencing the "return" of nature as a force that is literally pushing us indoors. We are back to a primordial fear. The accumulative blindness of the modern world, propelled by scientific technology, took the script too far. Nature had to find a way to tell human beings to back off.

In the last frame of the film, a girl is lying down, her head resting on a table, while a film plays on the monitor and trees sway outside the window. There is an uncanny peace in the frame.

Rome on the Balcony

Saturday, April 11

I WOKE UP LATE AS USUAL AND MADE TEA. THE SUN IS HOT TODAY. I had to take my elbows off the terrace parapet the moment I placed them there. I was looking out for the fruit seller to buy apples and bananas. But I found the snooty vegetable seller, instead. He had been obstructive the last time I spoke with him, and hesitant to sell me the green peas I wanted. His tomatoes were of good quality. There is a more amiable vegetable vendor who keeps his handcart right below my building. He only comes in the evening now, every other day. The handcarts are dependent on customers in these buildings. But everyone has stocked up, and we don't buy every day as we did before. The vendors also depend on passing trade, and people returning from work in the evenings. Both those possibilities are now removed, so the vendors have adjusted their schedules accordingly.

I DISCOVERED THE short film made by Mo Scarpelli for the *New Yorker*. *Rome, Closed City* (2020) was shot in Rome. Scarpelli is an Italian-American filmmaker, who documents life in the quarantined Italian capital as the pandemic surges across the country. It was released in March 2020. Scarpelli moved to Rome on March 1, and just managed to sign the lease of her apartment before the lockdown. She had neither a bed or a towel.[153] But she has managed to capture unforgettable images. With more than 18,000 deaths in Italy so far, a whole country waits to return to life.

In the film it seems as if people have suddenly abandoned the streets and sidewalks. The feeling of a great emptiness stares at you, eyeless, from every corner. The buildings are as empty as the cars, the cars as empty as the streets. The bus stops are as empty as the buses, the doors opening and closing with no one going in or out. There is a young woman on a swing outside a housing area, looking wistful, as if remembering someone from her childhood, or perhaps childhood itself. A child draws a rainbow, rain clouds, the sun and birds with chalk on the street. Nature is the metaphor of hope for children.

A bird pauses mid-air in front of a building, as if wondering what's wrong. It flies away. There are notes of caution taped to windows, about avoiding contact and maintaining distance. A small group of people stand outside a grocery store, each waiting for their turn to go in. They maintain a safe distance from one another. A young woman pulls down her mask and kisses her male companion on the lips, before going in.

Love is a risk that makes you feel safe. The word "safe" in the context of love always reminds me of these lines by A.K. Ramanujan, in the poem, 'Excerpts from a Father's Wisdom':

> If you wish to be safe in love
> court a mermaid.
> She's single-thighed.[154]

Back to the film: A wailing siren breaks the silence, piercing the landscape like a sinister bird-call. The bird sitting on the parapet above the river Tiber looks bewildered. The camera pauses for the bird to fly away. The nineteenth-century imperial figures of the Vitoriano building façade lie muted by time. Rome is watching itself on the balcony as the sun sets. The air is too risky.

ITALY WAS ONE of the countries that celebrated its health workers. I considered it a heart-warming gesture that people in Italy had gone onto their balconies on the afternoon of March 14 to give nationwide applause to doctors and nurses. I read that it had started with everyone singing the national anthem. People played the piano, trumpets, tambourines and violins, even pots and pans, to register their feelings in the middle of a mass house arrest. The whole episode was spontaneous, and it came from a mix of gratitude, sadness and anxiety, as well as a desire to express life amidst despair and confinement. It was a worthy response.

In contrast, in India, people clapped and clanged plates at an appointed time determined by the prime minister. People were following orders. The gesture lacked a genuine spirit of appreciation. The Indian middle class lacks motivation because their lives are focussed on the family, and their relationship with the world beyond that is purely an instrumental one. It is a tall task to think that a musical flash mob will perform on balconies as a mark of respect. They won't come to the balcony to decry the assault of doctors on the streets. These are people who want servitude, and to be told of their responsibilities by men in power.

Even a deadly virus cannot bring any change to their lives. They resist everything except privilege.

DURING DINNER, RICHA was watching a musical programme on television. The Mariinsky Theatre's *Nutcracker* had a profound impact on her. "The many senses this music lights up," she said, "we're moved by it... If only it were for everyone to enjoy — that truly is our Achilles heel." The arts, she believed, "help us transcend our pettiness." It may be true for those who are genuinely moved and inspired by it. She had also recently watched a stage production of Manganiyars music at the National Centre for the Performing Arts. The Manganiyars are Muslim folk artists from the region of the Thar Desert in Rajasthan. The programme made her think. "The folk performers were in show-boxes, instead of sitting together," she said, "choreographed for the consumption of city people."

Artists from remote regions undergo this artifice in the city. These designs are a product of a bizarre mindset: Nothing must be allowed to remain simple. Music from the rural world must be consumed and commodified on a stage that cannot resemble its natural setting. Thus, the rural is eulogised and forgotten at the same time. Such are the paradoxes of the connoisseur of culture in the city.

Dilshad Mohammad, Yannis Ritsos & Jafar Panahi

Sunday, April 12

THE DAY STARTED LATE AS USUAL. RICHA GOT FRUIT AND CURD from the grocer, so I could have bananas for breakfast, with tea. We had a dozen banana tree plants in our garden in Assam when I was a child. It was the "jahaji" variety, also known as the Dwarf Cavendish. Sometimes for fear of worms the bunch or the stem had to be cut off and brought home long before the bananas were close to ripening. Each banana was marked with slaked lime to make it ripen faster. It was magical to see the bananas change colour so quickly once a small mark of slaked lime was added to the skin with a finger. But the strategy used to backfire as the bananas ripened at such a fast pace, we could not eat them quick enough. So, father would distribute them among the neighbours. I remember once, when he handed a few overripe bananas to the aunt next door, I blurted out, "You know, he kept the better ones for us."

It embarrassed them both. My father apologised. She told him to ignore my provocative remark and thanked him. The story was often repeated among my family and neighbours and became something of a legend.

AFTER LUNCH, MY attention was drawn to a disturbing story. The story was a few days old, but a detailed report was only published today.[155] A thirty-seven-year-old man, Dilshad Mohammad, took his life on April 5. Hailing from a district in Himachal Pradesh, Mohammad had been accused by the people in his village of spreading the coronavirus, because he had offered a lift on his scooter to two men who had attended the Tablighi Jamaat event at Delhi's Nizamuddin. He tested negative. But it didn't stop the villagers holding him responsible for putting people at risk. Mohammad had driven the two men to the highway at the behest of the village maulvi. There was a strict lockdown in place. Mohammad's fraternal act was considered an act against the village. His loyalties were questioned.

Let us look at the ethical question involved in the incident. By helping the two men, Mohammad stood by his fraternal feelings, but risked his fraternal relationship with the village. One may argue it was an error of judgement. But the judgement itself was based on caring and goodwill. Mohammad preferred to err in helping the two Muslim men, rather than not do anything at all and stay at home.

To put it another way, Mohammad was confronted by a choice between principle and rule. Ambedkar explains the distinction in *Annihilation of Caste*:

> Doing what is said to be good by virtue of a rule, and doing good in the light of a principle, are two different things. The principle may be wrong, but the act is *conscious and responsible*. The rule may be right, but the act is *mechanical*. A religious act may not be a correct act but must at least be a responsible act. To permit of

this responsibility, Religion must mainly be a matter of principles only. It cannot be a matter of rules. [156] [My emphasis]

Mohammad could have chosen not to help the men, and mechanically adhered to the rules he was expected to follow. A religion (or in this case, a society) that does not appreciate principles but lives by rules alone, 'degenerates,'[157] according to Ambedkar.

It is true that people need to stay at home and not risk endangering others in potentially spreading the coronavirus. But to respond to the human calamity we also need doctors, nurses and health workers to care for patients and conduct tests. These women and men risk their lives to carry out their duty. They follow the *principle* of medical service amid a global emergency. Mohammad followed his principle as a human being.

AFTER LUNCH, I picked up a copy of Yannis Ritsos' *Diaries of Exile*. It comprises of poems that Ritsos had written while detained at a centre for political prisoners. Ritsos was a communist and was held at the German-run camp in the village of Kontopouli, during the Axis occupation of Greece in the fall of 1948. The poems are short. Ritsos uses simple images masterfully, with occasional, laconic expressions, to convey the mood of desolation and uncertainty in confinement. 'The night had no hours,'[158] he writes on November 6. The line makes me think of the days and nights in lockdown. Time in any form of confinement dissolves into a suffocating timelessness. Ritsos' time and our time form an arc of similarity.

A friend called later that night from Cambridge, Massachusetts. She said she had lost all sense of time. She used to wear a watch, but no longer did. In my case, I feel that time has lost its uniformity. It is suddenly 12pm, or 5pm, or 2.30am. But the time between morning and afternoon, or between afternoon and evening, or between dinner and midnight, feels endless. I have stopped believing the time registered on my mobile phone. When the night has no hours, the clock has no hands.

Like my friend in Cambridge and many others, I stopped wearing a watch a long time ago. I have a Titan with a black strap, gifted by my mother. It lies in a cupboard somewhere. I wish to wear it again someday. The humidity of the Delhi summer never made me want to wear a watch, while in winter one wears so many clothes that arms are heavy already. Even if I was to wear a watch, likely I'd forget it was there. It is easier to check the time on the phone.

The next lines in Ritsos' *Diaries* also catch my attention:

We don't need to shave so often.
The days and the hands move slowly. We're used to it.[159]

Life was slow like in Ritsos' poem, even though not as harsh. I looked sombre, reflective and sad. I wondered when I will feel like shaving again.

On November 13, Ritsos writes, 'Maybe tomorrow the old things will happen again. Nothing is certain.'[160]

In his later life, Ritsos was confined to a sanatorium for tuberculosis. Here his interest in Marxism grew. The element of patience and hope that quietly resides in Ritsos' poetry comes from having survived illness and political imprisonment alike.

Covid-19 won't disappear from our lives, even though cases may diminish, and the threat may become less palpable. We need to be cautious. Social distancing will become the new norm. Paranoia will guide our intimate relations. People will be scared to kiss or make love. The world until now was already running low on trust. The new biological scare will intensify our mutual alienation. The future is uncertain.

I WATCHED MY third film in lockdown: Jafar Panahi's *3 Faces* (2018). One of Iran's most influential film directors, Panahi remains defiant in the face of a ban imposed on his work by the Iranian government. *3 Faces* won the best screenplay award at Cannes.

The setting for *3 Faces* is a deeply patriarchal village. The film revolves around a young woman whose hopes of working in films after getting married comes to a standstill. The film aims to show that no one understands one another until they make the effort. It is another timely reminder in a world where people have less time and patience for each other, and prefer interacting as ghosts through technology. Language has lost its face. The film blurs the line between fiction and reality (docufiction), a genre and technique that Iranian filmmakers have mastered over the years. I found it to be closest to Kiarostami's sensibility. Kiarostami wrote the screenplay for Panahi's first film, *The White Balloon* (1995), and his controversial *Crimson Gold* (2003).

Panahi is important to remember in these times. He has

been making films illegally since 2011, when a court in Tehran passed a sentence to place him under house arrest and ban him from filmmaking. Panahi smuggled a film to France, which he made under house arrest that same year. *This Is Not a Film* (2011) was screened at the Cannes Film Festival. It shows Panahi in conversation with members of his family and his lawyer. He discusses the sentence imposed on him by the government and reflects on the craft of filmmaking.

Panahi also made two more films illegally, having been allowed to travel around the country. *Taxi* (2015) is exceptional, with a hidden camera placed above the dashboard. Making the film, Panahi pretended to be a cab driver, and documented his interactions with the various customers he takes through the city. When a friend and human rights lawyer recognises him, she offers him a flower. Panahi is a beacon; he teaches not only filmmakers, but all artists, how to work under constraint and uphold the spirit of life. Creativity is often a product of the struggle between art and life, which is also the case under lockdown. Perhaps the most striking aspect of these films lies in Panahi's assertion that if confinement against artistic freedom is legal, art has no other recourse but work through illegal means to exist.

Of Sleep, Dreams & Insomnia

Monday, April 13

I DECIDED TO GO BACK TO SLEEP SHORTLY AFTER WAKING UP AND having my breakfast of tea and biscuits. It reminded me of my days in JNU.

JNU's hostels are named after rivers. And they all suffer from a shortage of water. The irony was never clearer than in summer. But in winter, sleep was more sought after than bathing. I remember a Sunday morning in Brahmaputra hostel. Bidhan and I finished our breakfast at the mess, with eggs, bread and coffee. Coffee was never my favoured drink. I grew up in Assam, with the flavour of Assam and Darjeeling tea. Father preferred a 60–40 mix: 60 Darjeeling and 40 Assam, since Darjeeling was lighter in flavour. He had endless cups of tea during the day. The few times I visited him in his office, he always had a cup of tea on the table.

In Bengali homes, at least among the East-Bengali middle-class refugee homes in Assam, there was a strange prohibition: children were not allowed to have tea. Tea was considered addictive, hence restricted to adults. During school exams, when I needed a hot drink to study, I was given Horlicks and Viva but never tea. Sipping endless cups of tea in JNU, I used to recall the naïve paranoia of Bengalis, even when it came to something as innocuous as tea.

On Sundays we were offered coffee instead of tea in the hostel.

I did not mind coffee on winter mornings. After we walked out of the mess after breakfast, I asked Bidhan what his plans for the day were. He gave me the look he always did when he had something profoundly amusing on his mind.

"Do you know what the best time to sleep is during the day?" he asked, matter of factly.

I shook my head.

With an air of assurance, he told me. "It is right after breakfast, sir."

I should have guessed. Only the laziest man in the world would offer such an insight. I felt obliged to take him at his word and followed him in another round of blissful sleep till lunch.

I did the same thing this morning. I remember waking up twice in the early hours to check a message on my phone. I generally avoid this practice and put my phone on silent at bedtime. But sometimes it happens for no discernible reason. We take pleasure in technology being at our command, but we forget the fact that technology has enslaved us.

In my sleep, the one after breakfast, I dreamt of my old mathematics teacher, Maria Lewis. If I had known about the German poet, Rainer Maria Rilke, at school, I would have asked Lewis if his mother — like Rilke's — had given him the name Maria because she had expected a daughter. I would also have asked if she made him wear skirts as a child, like Rilke's mother did. In the dream, I was in my old central government school near the railway station in Maligaon I was looking for Mr Lewis (we used to address him "sir", as per convention) as dusk was falling, and so there were long shadows in the school corridor. I was looking in one empty room after another. It was the wrong time to look for my teacher because school had been over at 3.30pm. But I was dreaming, and dreams are not obliged to follow rules.

I wonder how dreams create plots, like we see in films. Dreams are our first teachers in art. I am sure the first idea of fiction and cinema appeared because of dreams. In dreams, the idea is transformed into image. Cinema had to wait for technology to invent itself. Fiction is always written like a dream that one recollects through the form of story. Being "lost" in a story is to experience a dreamlike sensation. Cinema is of course much like a dream: observed in a darkened theatre, one dreams through the film and makes private associations.[161] Cinema is dreaming with open eyes. Cinema is a paradoxical state of dreaming: to dream privately in public.

Dreams are more private than sex. When we dream, we are totally alone. It also guarantees our freedom. No power can rob us of our dreams.

There was no sight of Mr Lewis. Then I remembered a room where he might be and peeped in. He was there, at his desk, writing. He said he would be fifteen more minutes and then could leave. He added we could go to a place and sit like last time. But which place? Where? I had no idea and did not ask. He gave me a notebook. What was I supposed to write? Did Mr Lewis appear in my dream because he wanted something from me? Did he want to know if I remembered him? Did he want to know what I thought of him after all these years? I wondered whether I come into his dreams, too.

We did not leave the room. Mr Lewis continued to work at his desk. I wondered some more about what to write but couldn't write anything because I wanted to talk to him. I continued to wait for him to finish his work. He never did, however, and then the dream ended. I wondered what the dream meant, if indeed dreams mean anything.

As a teacher Mr Lewis never raised a hand, or his voice. We had confrontations initially because I was a mischievous student and loved playing pranks. Mr Lewis wanted order. Finally, on reaching tenth grade, we became friends.

As a boy, I respected elders who showed an element of respect towards me. I dismissed those who only knew how to impose humourless authority over children. Many years later I felt vindicated by the Russian writer Vladimir Rozanov:

The rule that *children should respect their parents and that parents should love their children* should be reversed. It is the parents who must *respect their children* — respect their strange little worlds and their excitable nature quick to feel hurt at any moment. Children should only *love* their parents, and they will certainly love them when they feel they are being respected.[162]

Rozanov makes complete sense. Love does not need schooling. Respect is what you learn from people who set examples. I read it too late, when I was at university. I almost cried. If I knew these words while at school, I would have read them aloud as part of my "Thought for the Day" in morning assembly. I would have also written it and pinned it above my desk at home.

A classmate and I decorated Mr Lewis's house with coloured paper and fairy lights at Christmas. I always loved Christmas, although sadly did not have a Christian friend and so never got invited to share in the festivities. I always wanted to fall in love with a Christian girl. I thought of going to mass but never did, due again to lack of company. But I still have fond memories of being woken up at dawn on Christmas day as parties would pass by my house, wearing colourful shawls, playing the guitar and singing carols. I would wave at them from my veranda and wish them well. They would reciprocate with a smile.

I had an affair with a Bengali Christian woman in Kolkata, during my MPhil days in JNU. We walked the crowded Rashbehari Avenue, and talked on a bench beside the lake at Rabindra Sarobar. I brought her flowers. She gifted me the fragrance of an empty room. The affair started in summer but never reached Christmas.

Mr Lewis used to treat us to chicken and plain dosa cooked by his aged mother. On the brink of my breakup with a girl in school, I asked him if I could meet her at his place. We did not have any place to be together, so that we could sit and talk. Meeting outside was risky in a small town where you might easily bump into someone who knew you. The older generation of middle-class railway employees followed conservative social mores. Their marriages were fixed through traditional rules that included caste laws. Premarital romance was seen as a corrupting influence, like popular cinema and western ideas. The romantic sensibility of my generation was partly shaped by the rebellious love stories in popular films. Hindi cinema celebrates premarital romance, often between lovers across language and religious divides. The themes of these films are influenced by the epic stories of love like *Laila-Majnun* (a seventh-century love story of Arabic origin), *Shirin-Farhad* (a twelfth-century love story of Persian origin), and *Heer-Ranjha* (a Punjabi love ballad written in 1766 by Waris Shah). The tradition of playback singing in popular cinema, where lovers convey the many moods and travails of love, also impacted us deeply. Western literature and culture shaped our erotic sensibilities. We were breaking traditionalist norms, and felt Rimbaud's decisive proclamation in our eclectic, postcolonial world: 'It is necessary to be absolutely modern.'[163]

Mr Lewis was Christian with a liberal sensibility, but his mother belonged to an older and more conservative generation. He agreed reluctantly. That evening, at his house, I waited and waited. She never turned up. I felt embarrassed.

Mr Lewis had asked me to meet him the next day. Sitting in the empty school library, he said, simply, life is not all fairy lights, or Christmas.

I WOKE UP and made tea. I checked the world news. An article in the *New York Times* covered the outbreak of wildfires in Chernobyl, which had raised concerns about a possible increase in radiation. After the 1986 disaster, around the nuclear power plant was "the Zone of Alienation,"[164] an eighteen-mile radius of land fenced off with barbed wire.

In his movie, *Stalker*, there is a scene where a telephone rings in the middle of a heated discussion taking place in a delapidated building. The telephone is answered and a confused exchange takes place, the caller evidently expecting to have got through to a clinic. Perhaps this is what the building once was? The call is a haunting reminder for the audience of the violent disruption that has occurred between people and place. Like the Zone, Chernobyl exists as a living sore, a protected area that is still exposed to dangerous accidents.

The night arrived without notice, and passed slowly, like a ship from another century. If you disconnect your ties with the world for a while, you can begin to inhabit other times. The night is full of questions: When will I see mother? When will I take Richa to my old hometown, and the Kamakhya Temple? Nostalgia is biting my flesh, passing like a slow ship over my sleepy eyes, and the unanswerable questions continue. When will I visit the Safdarjung Tomb, with my bottled water and fruit? Have tea and snacks at Qahwa? When will I walk the cobblestoned lanes of Khan Market like a well-dressed ghost looking for attention? When will I see the gentle sales assistant at Bahri Sons? When will I sit with Abir in the Parsi café at Khan Market, and have masala tea with potato fries?

Some places, like times, do not exist anymore. I remember visiting the bookstore, Bookworm, at Connaught Place, one morning around fifteen years ago. There I met an old JNU friend, Andaleeb, now in the employment of the railway. He was taking the evening train back to Mumbai, where he lived. We collected the books we had been searching for and decided to revisit old times over beer at Volga, a red-carpeted, delightfully cheap and laidback bar. I occasionally frequented the place, but my ties with it were intense. A friend once called me in the afternoon. As he spoke, I interrupted him, "Are you outside Volga?" He was taken aback,

"How do you know?" I had caught the sound of the flautist in the background. The man sold flutes outside Volga. No other flautist in the city played that poignant song of separated lovers, like he did.

Neither Bookworm, nor Volga, exist today.

Some people, too, like places and times, do not exist anymore. My dear friend, Jawahar, died in London in January 2020. The news caused a tremor in the heart. He did not sing, but a lot of music flowed in him. He was thirsty for the bitter salt of the sea and drank like a fish. Jawahar was always at sea with his emotions and kept silent about them. Some years earlier, I had sent him a poem about our time at university. His reply suggested that he was sinking with the weight of memory: 'As breathtaking a read as the final breath.' In winter last year, he came home, and we met after many years apart. The chicken curry I made for him was, he said, better than anything he had eaten in all of London. We toasted the past with wine. We couldn't know that we were collecting a final souvenir.

THE MIND IS at sea, confronting a sea of questions. Sleep is on the other side. The memories of childhood are as close as the memory of last night. I remember lines from Marina Tsvetaeva's poem, 'Insomnia':

> Who sleeps at night? No one is sleeping.
> In the cradle a child is screaming.
> An old man sits over his death, and anyone
> young enough talks to his love, breathes
> into her lips, looks into her eyes.

Once asleep who knows if we'll wake again?
We have time, we have time, we have time to sleep![165]

The social traffic of the digital world reminds us that the world never truly sleeps. The world stopped sleeping with the parallel world of the internet, and the digital insomnia of lockdown suggests a deeper crisis. It is not just everyday life that is under lockdown; the immediate future is hazy and uncertain. The future is under lockdown as well. The idea of time has vanished.

Seconds, minutes, hours (of work, leisure or travel) are suddenly no longer reliable. Space and time are no longer synchronous, but monotonous and constant. Time doesn't move. The world and time are no longer as we know them. In this radically altered time, we suddenly have a lot of time for ourselves. But it is a time without numbers, without hours and dates. Time is sun and shadow. There is fear at every step, in every touch.

Marina Tsvetaeva beautifully plays on the paradox. *We have time, we have time, we have time to sleep!* There is enough time at our disposal for sleep. But we find no time to sleep. Something keeps us awake. We want the night to deliver us outside the time that has locked us in. We sink into the night with our eyes open, not risking the dawn.

Then suddenly, without warning, sleep will arrive like a speeding goods train in the depth of night, and carry us off to an unknown destination.

To Cross or Not Cross the Line

Tuesday, April 14

I WOKE UP A LITTLE AFTER THE PRIME MINISTER'S ADDRESS TO THE nation. News was already out in the media that the lockdown would be extended. Now it was official: the lockdown was extended to May 3.

It is one thing to support the government's decision and agree that extending the lockdown in this emergency is necessary. It is another to live it and see one's fears and anxieties extended for an uncertain number of days. It is one thing to agree with the lockdown because it technically puts your life in less danger. But it is another to remember that there are lives incomparably less privileged than yours, and those who need money to survive and eat.

You are caught between what French thinker Michel Foucault calls 'care of the self'[166] and caring for others. In a capitalist society, caring for oneself is a strict set of habits: fitness, food and beauty regimes that involve time in the gym, maintaining a health food diet, and visiting the beauty salon or parlour. It is a range of activities with purely material obligations.

A journalist joked on Twitter that a haircut should be included as an essential service. Foucault tells us that in the Hellenistic period (after Plato), the 'care of the self' included writing. Writing treatises, letters, notebooks and confessions were modes of self-discovery. It produced writers as varied as Marcus Aurelius, Saint Augustine and Jean-Jacques Rousseau. In India, we have Gandhi and Nehru, among others. They wrote what is considered the modern confessional, the autobiography. Though writers have lived and written in poverty with meagre means, writing is still considered a privilege, something for the elite and those who have the luxury to avoid other forms of labour. The meaning of writing, however, cannot be evaluated simply in sociological terms. There is an unexpected quality in the expression of all art where something new is produced.

Writing can offer something new. Often, new times provoke new thoughts and genres in writing. The time in which we are living is new. We are in the middle of a new dystopia, the time of the Anthropocene, the deepening and widening shadow of fascism in democracies, and the rise of religious terrorism. Amid all this, Covid-19 has arrived with a new state (and sense) of emergency. It has ripped apart the boundaries of political reason — nation, religion, race and caste — and the boundaries of what we narcissistically call "identity", by levelling the distinctions of identity so that they don't matter anymore. In the eyes — and viruses — of nature, our differences don't matter. We are a species under threat. But pandemics have never prevented humans from being stupid about their identity.

Death — even the spectacle of mass death during war and pandemics — hasn't given pause to the world, that it might ponder on its ethical failings and reimagine life. The rule books and privileges are too ingrained in society for people to flaunt them. People would rather falter on what comes easily, rather than attempt a new, more humane failure.

A STRANGE EPISODE keeps reappearing in my mind when I think of this issue. We had gone to visit my paternal aunt in a place called Barasat in Kolkata's North 24 Parganas. Her late husband (my father's elder brother) was an editor of a bimonthly newspaper, *Shahor Theke Dure* (*Away from the City*), which he ran for eighteen years. One of the main issues tackled by the newspaper was the forced occupation of land. He was a patriarch who would irritate the schoolboy me with English grammar. (Growing up, I met many Bengalis who were obsessed with grammar and ignored the flowering of language. The journey of language does not lie in grammar. Grammar is simply a road sign that you follow to stay on course.) That evening in Barasat I met my aunt for the last time. She was in bed, reduced to skin and bones. She shared her tribulations, which included the difficulty she had in reaching the bathroom. She complained that her younger son and his family remained upstairs and did not care for her. Then she spoke of a robbery that had recently taken place, which had resulted in the loss of her jewellery. She cursed the thief and mourned her jewels. It was a pathetic and ironic sight. This old woman, whose days were clearly limited, was unrelenting; she craved her jewellery like someone expecting to wear it at the next wedding in town.

The jewels held a special place in her memory, but they did not matter to her life at that point. She should have considered the theft an act of providence. It served her son right for not looking after her. The thief was a character out of a fable. He served a form of justice, taking from the old woman the jewels she no longer had a need for, as well as from the son destined to inherit them but who didn't deserve them.

It wasn't the jewellery itself but the fetish of jewellery that had a deep hold on her psyche. Jewellery is a metaphor for identity. It is an empty (surplus) value of identity, with which we exploit (and hoodwink) ourselves.

THINKING ABOUT THE invisible but firm line that has been between home and the world, my mind goes back to March 24, when the prime minister said, "Today's decision of countrywide lockdown has drawn a "Lakshman Rekha" around the door of your house."[167]

It is interesting to note that among the many Ramayanas, it is the Bengali version of the *Ramayana* written by the fifteenth-century poet, Krittibas Ojha, called *Krittivasi Ramayana* that contains the only reference to "Lakshman Rekha". In the story, the exiled king, Ram's younger brother, Lakshman, draws the line (in the shape of an arc) for Sita as a mark of protection. Sita is tempted by kindness to cross the line when the demon king, Ravan, disguised as a beggar, asks her for alms. Once Sita steps over the line, Ravan takes her away by force. This leads to war between Ram and Ravan. The story has stood as a metaphor for patriarchal order and law, couched under the discourse of (a woman's) dharma. The "Lakshman Rekha" is placed at the heart of the epic to impart a moral lesson: temptation of any kind leads to danger, and resisting temptation is the mark of dharma. Sita's crossing the line was a moment of gullibility that was necessary to draw the moral of good winning over evil. The line of obedience had to be trespassed to reestablish virtuous order. The moral agony against crossing the line is contradictory: You need the gullible act you are agonized by, and you are agonized, in turn, by that gullibility.

To cross or not cross the line has been the moral question. But human freedom is not possible without risking the line (of morality) that controls you. If the beggar asking for alms was not disguised with wicked intentions, the motivation behind Sita's crossing of the line would have been acceptable. Her act of kindness was ruined by someone else's deceit. The point is: the motivations of ethical life, gullible or not, can't be overruled by an aberration. The epic nature of the epidemic does not merely demand obedience from a nation's citizens, but also places responsibilities on the state. Nothing about the government's responsibility was spelt out by the prime minister.

Reports of domestic abuse emerged from various parts of the world, including India. No virus can activate reflection on oneself. There is a firm line drawn against it.

The extension of the lockdown was followed by news of migrant workers gathering in their thousands at the Bandra station in Mumbai. These were workers from Bihar, Uttar Pradesh, and Assam among others. While the government focused on the lockdown, the working class was worried about its daily meals and uncertain livelihood. A state of confusion was inevitable. There can't be a lack of initiative when people need to know they won't go hungry. The police lathi charged on the crowd that had gathered. Everything begins and ends, for the state and its partisan television networks, with law and order.

TAKE THE CASE of Lisa Jose,[168] a nurse in a Delhi hospital. She discovered on April 4 that she had contracted coronavirus from an infected doctor. Jose was eight months pregnant and had to quarantine herself at the hospital she worked in. The next day, walking to the ambulance that came to take her away, Jose found herself the subject of videos being taken by her neighbours on their phones. In her words, "I felt like a criminal being taken away... What wrong had I done? I only did my duty."[169]

What wrong had Lisa Jose committed? Her greatest crime, in the eyes of her jaundiced neighbours, was falling prey to the virus. The karma theory of causality that equates birth, fate and virtue (or the lack of it) is fertile ground for prejudice. If someone catches a disease, it is a result of a bad or wrong action committed in a previous life. If the person happens to be you, or a family member, the logic is conveniently discarded. Not so if the person turns out to be a neighbour.

Jose was made to feel she was a wrongdoer. She caught the virus and was unceremoniously cast out. The collective gaze of the neighbours preyed on her. The myth of collective virtue abides by the power to humiliate others. In such a society, people who live with empathy and love live outside these collective codes of fake and violent morality.

In India, the idea of the 'care of the self' as an individual ethic is present only in a limited sense. Self-care needs a certain self-knowledge and practice that may lead to spiritual and ethical transformation. That possibility is mediated (and interrupted) by fixed social notions. Caste and religious rules discourage enquiry. One needs to create one's own (social) space in order to pursue enquiry, which is why young people who want to think on their own must live on their own and escape the stranglehold of the family. The family transmits germs of prejudice across generations. No natural virus can eradicate this social virus.

There is a sense of entitlement to not caring about others, especially if it disturbs fixed notions of deference and superiority. The self is a "rekha" (boundary). Everyone beyond the line is a potential and harmful demon. Then there is the other fear — of touch.

Social distancing becomes a norm in the face of this paranoia. We exchange money for goods with workers who bring essential goods to our doorsteps, or those who hand them to us in grocery shops. Along with goods and money, you also exchange your fears. Queues outside stores for essential items have people standing within circles that are marked to help keep safe distance. Our distances have become precise, like our fears. Everyone looks like an alien from another planet, frozen and muted by a strange lack of communication. There is nothing to communicate between people who suffer the same fear.

The new emergency warns against touch and advocates 'social distancing'. The new norm, or law, is based on a biological fear. It breaks through all social hierarchies. Everyone lives in the shadow of their own fear. The virus lives in that shadow. The virus is the shadow.

Untouchability is the bane of upper caste lives. If you create a world of touchable and untouchable people and objects, you create an internal design for paranoia. The idea of the "rekha" works here too, where you daily pass through (and avoid) numerous lines that run between the touchable and the untouchable. These lines demarcate the shadowy zone between self-caring, and being uncaring towards others. Touch is outside the sphere of care.

As a species we have the unique ability to exaggerate real dangers in our imagination. The virus is real, but our fear blows it out of proportion. Every passing person might be carrying the virus. The virus is everywhere, in our eyes and in our minds, in everything we touch, in everything we avoid touching. The virus has consumed our collective imagination. It has distanced people from one another. The virus has created the paranoia of proximity. We fear other bodies. We fear our own bodies. We realise our bodies are porous and vulnerable. The act of washing hands with soap or sanitizer for twenty seconds, avoiding touching our face, makes us wary of our body. We must be saved from others and ourselves, and if nothing else the pandemic has taught us that nothing can be taken for granted. To be careful, we must take care. We are asked to touch *carefully*.

To touch or not to touch has been the central predicament in the lives of Hindus. Untouchability is part of the norm, or law, of Hindu life. Journalist Jeya Rani writes, that 'the caste virus is... an ever-present epidemic spread by touchable/rich India'.[170] Caste is an epidemic based on social distancing, whereas today we practise social distancing *because* there is an epidemic. Despite the reversible nature of their difference, the casualty in both cases is touch.

It is better to die of touch, than to die untouched.

Select bibliography

Alexievich, Svetlana, *Chernobyl Prayer: Voices from Chernobyl*, trans. Anna Gunin and Arc Tait. Penguin Classics, 2016.
Ambedkar, Babasaheb, 'Annihilation of Caste: With a Reply to Mahatma Gandhi,' in *Dr. Babasaheb Ambedkar, Writings and Speeches, Volume 1*. Government of Maharashtra, 1979.
Arendt, Hannah, 'Thinking and Moral Considerations', in *Responsibility and Judgement*. Schocken Books, 2005.
Barthes, Roland, *A Lover's Discourse: Fragments*, trans. Richard Howard. Hill and Wang, 1978.
Baudelaire, Charles, *Intimate Journals*, trans. Christopher Isherwood. Dover Publications, 2006.
——, *Selected Writings on Art and Literature*. Penguin, 1972.
Bellow, Saul, *Herzog*. Penguin Classics, 2003.
Belting, Hans, *Face and Mask: A Double History*, trans. Thomas S. Hansen and Abby J. Hansen. Princeton University Press, 2017.
Camus, Albert, *The Plague*, trans. Stuart Gilbert. Modern Library, 1948.
Canby, Vincent, 'Satyajit Ray's Moving "Distant Thunder": The Cast,' *New York Times*, 2 October 1973.
Cavafy, C.P., *Collected Poems*, trans. Edmund Keeley and Philip Sherrard. Chatto & Windus, 1998.
Cioran, E.M., *A Short History of Decay*. Quartet Books, 1990.
Darwish, Mahmoud, 'Like a Mysterious Incident,' in *The Butterfly's Burden*, trans. Fady Joudah. Copper Canyon Press, 2007.
Defoe, Daniel, *A Journal of the Plague Year*. Modern Library, 2001.
Dickinson, Emily, "'Hope' is the Thing with Feathers,' in *Complete Poems of Emily Dickinson*, edited by Thomas H. Johnson. The Belknap Press of Harvard University Press, 1955.
——, *Selected Poems*, edited by Stanley Appelbaum. Dover Publications, 1990.
Dostoevsky, Fyodor, *Demons*, trans. Robert A. Maguire. Penguin Classics, 2008.
Eliot, T.S., *The Complete Poems and Plays: 1909-1950*. Harcourt Brace and Company, 1971.

Fuentes, Carlos, *Diana: The Goddess Who Hunts Alone*, trans. Alfred Macadam. Bloomsbury, 1996.

Gandhi, M.K., *An Autobiography or the Story of My Experiments with Truth*, trans. Mahadev Desai. Penguin, 2018.

Gide, André, *Journals (Volume 2: 1914-1927)*, trans. Justin O'Brien. University of Illinois Press, 2000.

Hall, Stuart; Held, David; Hubert, Don; Thompson, Kenneth (eds), *Modernity: An Introduction to Modern Societies*. Wiley-Blackwell, 1996.

Kafka, Franz, *The Diaries of Franz Kafka: 1910-1913, Volume 1*, edited by Max Brod, trans. Joseph Kresh. Schocken Books, 1948.

Kundera, Milan, *Immortality*, trans. Peter Kussi. Grove Weidenfeld, 1990.

——, *Slowness*, trans. Linda Asher. HarperCollins, 1996.

——, *The Book of Laughter and Forgetting,* trans. Aaron Asher. Harper Perennial, 1996.

Mahapatra, Jayanta, *The Whiteness of Bone*. Penguin Viking, 1992.

Mandelstam, Osip, *Complete Poetry of Osip Emilevich Mandelstam*, trans. Burton Raffel and Alla Burago. State University of New York Press, 1973.

Márquez, Gabriel García, *Living to Tell the Tale*, trans. Edith Grossman. Alfred A. Knopf, 2003.

——, *The Last Interview and Other Conversations*. Melville House Publishing, 2015.

——, *Love in the Time of Cholera*, trans. Edith Grossman. Penguin, 1998.

Marx, Karl, and Engels, Friedrich, *Economic and Philosophical Manuscripts of 1844 and the Communist Manifesto*, trans. Martin Milligan. Prometheus Books, 1988.

Marx, Karl, *The Communist Manifesto*, edited by Joseph Katz, trans. Samuel Moore. Pocket Books, 1964.

Nietzsche, Friedrich, *Beyond Good and Evil*, trans. Walter Kaufman. Random House, 1966.

Nirala, Suryakant Tripathi, *A Life Misspent*, trans. Satti Khanna. Harper Perennial, 2016.

Outka, Elizabeth, *Viral Modernism: The Influenza Pandemic and Interwar Literature*. Columbia University Press, 2020.

Paz, Octavio, 'Dostoevsky: The Devil and the Ideologue,' in *On Poets and Others*. Arcade Publishing, 1990.

——, *The Collected Poems: 1957-1987*, edited by/trans. Eliot Weinberger. Indus, 1992.

——, *The Labyrinth of Solitude*. Penguin, 1985.

Pessoa, Fernando, *The Book of Disquiet*, edited by Maria José de Lancastre, trans. Margaret Jull Costa. Hachette India, 2010.

Ramanujan, A.K., *Collected Poems*. Oxford India Paperbacks, 1997.

Rimbaud, Arthur, *Collected Poems*, trans. Martin Sorell. Oxford University Press, 2001.

Ritsos, Yannis, *Diaries of Exile*. Archipelago Books, 2013.

Robinson, Andrew, *Satyajit Ray: The Inner Eye*. University of California Press, 1989.

Rozanov, Vasily, *The Apocalypse of Our Time and other writings*, trans. Robert Pyne and Nikita Romanoff. Praeger Publishers, 1977.

Satchidanandan, K., *While I Write*. HarperCollins, 2011.

Sebald, W.G., *Across the Land and the Water: Selected Poems 1964-2001*. Hamish Hamilton, 2011.

Shakespeare, William, *Othello*, edited by E.A.J. Honigmann. Thomson Learning, 1997.

Shukla, Vinod Kumar, *Hari Ghas ki Chhapar Wali Chopri aur Bauna Pahad*. Rajkamal, 2011.

Snow, Edward, A., 'Loves of Comfort and Despair: A Reading of Shakespeare's Sonnet 138,' *English Literary History*, 47:3 (Autumn 1980), 462-83.

Sontag, Susan, *On Photography*. Penguin, 2002.

Stavans, Ilan, *Gabriel García Márquez: The Early Years*. Palgrave Macmillan, 2010.

Tagore, Rabindranath, 'Nationalism in the West,' in *Nationalism*. Penguin, 2009.

Thoreau, David, *Walden; or, Life in the Woods*. Princeton University Press, 1989.

Tsvetaeva, Marina, *Selected Poems*, trans. Elaine Feinstein. Oxford University Press, 1971.

Weber, Max, *The Protestant Ethic and the Spirit of Capitalism*, trans. Talcott Parsons. Scribner, 1958.

Whitman, Walt, *Leaves of Grass*. Vintage Classics, 2019.

Woolf, Virginia, 'On Being Ill,' *The New Criterion: A Quarterly Review*, 4:1 (January 1926), 32-45.

——, *Mrs. Dalloway*. Harcourt, 2005.

Zbigniew, Herbert, *The Collected Poems: 1956–1998*, trans Alisa Valles. Ecco Press, 2008.

Filmography

Abbas Kiarostami, *24 Frames* (2017)
——, *Through the Olive Trees* (1994)
——, *Taste of the Cherry* (1997)
Bernard L. Kowalski, *Macho Callahan* (1970)
Ingmar Bergman, *Persona* (1966)
Jafar Panahi, *3 Faces* (2018)
——, *Crimson Gold* (2003).
——, *The White Balloon* (1995)
——, *This Is Not a Film* (2011)
Jean-Luc Godard, *Breathless* (1960)
Akira Kurosawa, *Dreams* (1990)
Mo Scarpelli, *Rome, Closed City* (2020)
Ritesh Batra, *Lunchbox* (2013)
——, *Photograph* (2019)
Satyajit Ray, *Pratidwandi/The Adversary* (1970)
——, *Aranyer Din Ratri/ Days and Nights in the Forest* (1970)
——, *Ashani Sanket/Distant Thunder* (1973)
——, *Ghare Baire/The Home and the World* (1985)
——, *Kanchenjunga* (1962)
——, *Kapurush/The Coward* (1985)
——, *Mahanagar/ The Big City* (1963)
——, *Pather Panchali/Song of the Little Road* (1955)
——, *Seemabaddha/Company Limited* (1971)
Sergei Eisenstein, *Battleship Potemkin* (1926)
Vishal Bharadwaj, *Haider* (2014)
Werner Herzog, *Meeting Gorbachev* (2018)

Notes

1 T.S Eliot, *The Complete Poems and Plays: 1909-1950* (Harcourt Brace and Company, 1971) p.22.
2 Ibid.
3 My translation.
4 Charles Baudelaire, *Selected Writings on Art and Literature* (Penguin, 1972), p.402.
5 Ibid., p.403.
6 According to Bentham, 'the happiness of the body politic' will depend on four 'subordinate objects — Subsistence. Abundance. Equality. Security.' Jeremy Bentham, *The Works of Jeremy Bentham (Part II)*, edited by John Bowring (William Tait, 1838), p.302.
7 Charles Baudelaire, *Intimate Journals*, trans. Christopher Isherwood (Dover Publications, 2006), p.31.
8 Albert Camus, *The Plague*, trans. Stuart Gilbert (Modern Library, 1948), p.75.
9 My translation.
10 Its source lies in the Protestant work ethic of the modern era, as Max Weber reminds us.
11 Eliot, *Complete Poems and Plays*, p.58.
12 From an article by Shri Mahadev Desai in Harijan. This article was subsequently reprinted as a preface to M.K. Gandhi, *Hind Swaraj* (Navajivan Publishing House, 1938), p.8.
13 Ibid.
14 Dileep Padgaonkar, 'An Area of Awakening: V.S. Naipaul in Conversation with Dileep Padgaonkar,' *Sunday Times of India*, 18 July 1993, pp.10-11.
15 Ibid.
16 Ibid.
17 I was reminded of Elian when I read of the tragic death of the three-year-old Syrian refugee boy, Alan Kurdi, who was drowned on 2 September 2015, attempting to reach the Greek island of Kos. Both incidents relate to the unforgettable lines in the poem, 'Home', by Somali-British

writer and poet, Warsan Shire, who wrote: 'no one puts their children in a boat / unless the water is safer than the land.' Refugees (including the beleaguered ones whose citizenship is currently questioned in Assam) die in land and water.

18 Gabriel García Márquez, *Love in the Time of Cholera*, trans. Edith Grossman (Penguin, 1988), p.111.

19 Ibid., p.112.

20 David Thoreau, *Walden; or, Life in the Woods* (Princeton University Press, 1989), p.90.

21 Milan Kundera, *Immortality*, trans. Peter Kussi (Grove Weidenfeld, 1990), p.74.

22 There is an interesting corollary to my comparison: a 1970 short story by Márquez titled, 'Death Constant beyond Love'.

23 Name changed.

24 Zack Wortman, 'Ernest Hemingway's Six-Word Sequels', *The New Yorker*, 11 September 2016, https://www.newyorker.com/humor/daily-shouts/ernest-hemingways-six-word-sequels

25 Prawesh Lama and Kainat Sarfaraz, 'Slippers on bed, anti-CAA protest at Shaheen Bagh continues amid coronavirus outbreak', *Hindustan Times*, 23 March 2020, https://www.hindustantimes.com/india-news/slippers-on-bed-shaheen-protests-on/story-OjGk6A1jOxrp6HfD4KCzGP.html

26 A.K. Ramanujan, *Collected Poems* (Oxford India Paperbacks, 1997), p.19.

27 Anon., 'PM Modi fears India will be pushed back by 21 years if lockdown not successful', *Business Today*, 24 March 2020, https://www.businesstoday.in/current/economy-politics/pm-modi-announces-21-day-lockdown-of-entire-country-from-12am/story/399118.html

28 Gabriel García Márquez, *Living to Tell the Tale*, trans. Edith Grossman (Alfred A. Knopf, 2003), p.3.

29 Rabindranath Tagore, 'Nationalism in the West,' in *Nationalism* (Penguin, 2009), p.34.

30 Ibid., p.42.

31 'Ringed with a scum of chicken-necked bosses / he toys with the tributes of half-men.' Osip Mandelstam, 'The Stalin Epigram', Poets.org, https://poets.org/poem/stalin-epigram

32 I am reminded of the English translation of a short poem by Vinod Kumar Shukla, 'In Nature':

And I, the city man,
separate from nature so
that I leave the tree behind and sit in the bus.
Sitting in the bus, I wish
that there were trees on both sides of the road.
In my room
I have hung a picture of an entire forest.
We carry the devastation of nature in our hearts.

(https://www.poetryinternational.org/pi/poet/12941/Vinod-Kumar-Shukla/en/tile). I am also reminded of Professor Jamsheed Akrami's question to the late Iranian filmmaker, Abbas Kiarostami, during a July 2001 interview in a documentary, *A Walk with Kiarostami*, that took place in Ireland. Akrami noted, "In most of your photographs, you seem to focus on a single element, like a lone boat, a lone bird, or a lone tree." Kiarostami replied, "But of course a single tree is more of a tree than a number of them." He narrates the story of a girl who asked her father to show her the forest. The father took her. When they reached it, he asked her daughter if she could see the forest. The child replied, "Yes, but there are so many trees that I can hardly see the forest." Kiarostami explains that one confronts a new concept — that of a forest — when faced by a large number of trees. But it was difficult for the girl to make that conceptual and linguistic leap. The forest is an abstract concept for the presence of many trees. (https://www.youtube.com/watch?v=KKoSoL_jIWE)

33 Paavo Haavikko, *Selected Poems*, edited and trans. Anselm Hollo (Cape Goliard Press, 1968).

34 J. Laughlin (ed.), *New Directions in Prose and Poetry 37* (New Directions Publications Corporation, 1978), p.171.

35 Milan Kundera, *The Book of Laughter and Forgetting,* trans. Aaron Asher (Harper Perennial, 1996), p.2.

36 There were nationwide protests against the Citizenship Amendment Act (CAA) after it was passed by the government on 12 December 2019. The New Year arrived with JNU students and professors attacked by masked right-wing goons on the evening of 5 January 2020. There was a

Citizens March in New Delhi against the JNU violence and the CAA, on 9 January. There was a Rousseau among the protestors, a smiling, middle-aged man, holding a placard: 'The power of the people is much stronger than the people in power.' There were numerous placards of Gandhi. The anti-CAA protests were interrupted by riots in Delhi on 23 February, in predominantly Muslim neighbourhoods of north-east Delhi. People of both communities — Muslims and Hindus — lost their lives.

37 W.G. Sebald, *Across the Land and the Water: Selected Poems 1964–2001* (Hamish Hamilton, 2011), p.81.

38 Fernando Pessoa, *The Book of Disquiet*, edited by Maria José de Lancastre, trans. Margaret Jull Costa (Hachette India, 2010), p.vii.

39 Ibid., p.2.

40 Vinod Kumar Shukla, *Hari Ghas ki Chhapar Wali Chopri aur Bauna Pahad* (Rajkamal, 2011), p.5 (my translation).

41 Camus, *The Plague*, p.229.

42 Álvaro de Campos, 'Deferral,' trans. Richard Zenith, *The Virginia Quarterly Review*, 72:2 (Spring 1996), p.302.

43 Ibid.

44 Kabir Agarwal, "Hunger Can Kill Us Before the Virus': Migrant Workers on the March During Lockdown,' *The Wire*, 27 March 2020, https://thewire.in/labour/coronavirus-lockdown-migrant-workers-walking-home

45 Mentioned on p.58 (in section Light the Candles).

46 Virginia Woolf, *Mrs. Dalloway* (Harcourt, 2005), p.3.

47 Ibid., p.12.

48 Ibid., p.13.

49 Virginia Woolf, 'On Being Ill,' *The New Criterion: A Quarterly Review*, 4:1 (January 1926), p.32.

50 Ibid.

51 Ibid., p.38.

52 Ibid.

53 Agha Shahid Ali, 'The Walled City: 7 Poems of Delhi,' in *In Memory of Begum Akhtar* (Writers Workshop, 1979), p.30. Thanks to my student and friend, Manan Kapoor, for referring me to the book.

54 'In Pablo Neruda's home, on the Pacific / coast, I remembered Yannis

Ritsos.' From 'Like a Mysterious Incident', in Mahmoud Darwish, *The Butterfly's Burden*, trans. Fady Joudah (Copper Canyon Press, 2007), p.307.
55 Walt Whitman, *Leaves of Grass* (Vintage Classics, 2019), p.350.
56 Jayanta Mahapatra, 'The Abandoned British Cemetery at Balasore, India', Michael Hulse and Simon Rae (eds.), *The 20th Century in Poetry* (Ebury Press, 1988), p.557.
57 Ibid.
58 Anon., 'Coronavirus lockdown: India grapples with migrant workers' exodus', *Al Jazeera*, 28 March 2020, https://www.aljazeera.com/news/2020/03/coronavirus-lockdown-india-grapples-migrant-workers-exodus-200328151304900.html
59 Herbert Zbigniew, *The Collected Poems: 1956-1998*, trans. Alisa Valles (Ecco Press, 2008), p.136.
60 When I visited Srinagar in September 2015 with a delegation of poets chosen by Sahitya Akademi (India's National Academy of Letters), I breathed an uneasy calm. I felt one false step could mean trouble. The air in Srinagar was like barbed wire. The noisy delights of the fish market, young people walking along the Dal Lake oblivious of time, the aroma of 'Kahwa' (a Kashmiri version of green tea that includes saffron, cinnamon, cloves, dried rose petals, cardamom and almonds) beside the Jhelum were reassuring. At Hazratbal, the pigeons were the same as those found in temples. When I read my poems at the university, the show of appreciation moved me. I forgot I was a stranger.
61 Anna Akhmatova, *Selected Poems*, trans. D.M. Thomas (Penguin, 1988), p.87.
62 Ibid., p.96.
63 Arthur Rimbaud, *Collected Poems*, trans. Martin Sorell (Oxford University Press, 2001), p.xvii.
64 Name changed.
65 Octavio Paz, 'Sunstone,' in *The Collected Poems: 1957-1987*, edited and trans. Eliot Weinberger (Indus, 1992), p.23.
66 For Marx, '*alienation* of the worker in his product means not only that his labor becomes an object, an *external* existence, but that it exists *outside him*, independently, as something alien to him.' (Karl Marx and

Friedrich Engels, *Economic and Philosophical Manuscripts of 1844 and the Communist Manifesto,* trans. Martin Milligan (Prometheus Books, New 1988), p.72). Such a worker, in Marx's conception, undergoes a double-alienation: he too is transformed into an *'alien* being' (p.79). Alienated from within and from (the product of) his own labour, the worker becomes the victim of a larger phenomenon where 'one man is estranged from the other, as each of them is from man's essential nature' (p.78) By essential nature, Marx suggests nature as 'sensuous' (p.111).

67 The everyday life of the traditional world in Europe 'before the Protestant Reformation... (was) punctuated by saints' days, fairs, pilgrimages, festivals, seasons of feasting'. It was replaced by a world led by 'rational forms of explanation'. This 'application of instrumental reason' to explain life (which meant maximizing efficiency and being economical, and pursuing rationally determined goals), is what Weber saw as a process of 'de-magification' (German: *Entzauberung der Welt*, also translated as 'the disenchantment of the world', a term Weber borrowed from Friedrich Schiller. This process is also understood as *'secularization'*. See Robert Bocock, 'The Cultural Formations of Modern Society,' in Stuart Hall, David Held, Don Hubert and Kenneth Thompson (eds), *Modernity: An Introduction to Modern Societies* (Wiley-Blackwell, 1996), p.175.

68 Tweet by Sara Jefry, 15 March 2020, https://twitter.com/sarajefry/status/1239265680253489153?lang=en

69 See Hans Belting's *Face and Mask: A Double History,* trans. Thomas S. Hansen and Abby J. Hansen (Princeton University Press, 2017).

70 Friedrich Nietzsche, *Beyond Good and Evil*, trans. Walter Kaufman (Random House, 1966), p.229.

71 A few weeks later, a photographer friend texted me to thank me and my friend again, for sending him the recipe. He said, "It was life-saving." I told Aman, he was no longer only a writer now, but a doctor too.

72 Michel De Montaigne, *The Complete Essays of Montaigne*, trans. Donald M. Frame (Stanford University Press, 1958), p.137.

73 Ibid.

74 Ibid.

75 Ibid., p.139.

76 Marx and Engels, *Communist Manifesto*, p.62.

77 Márquez, *Living to Tell the Tale*, p.106.
78 Anon, Ecclesiastes 3:1–8, Poets.org, https://poets.org/poem/ecclesiastes-31-8
79 Eliot, *Complete Poems and Plays,* pp.127–28.
80 Whan that Aprille with his shoures sote
    The droghte of Marche hath perced to the rote,
    And bathed every veyne in swich licour,
    Of which vertu engendred is the flour
    Geoffrey Chaucher, *The Canterbury Tales* (1387–1400), reader-friendly edition in modern spelling by Michael Murphy available at http://academic.brooklyn.cuny.edu/webcore/murphy/canterbury/2genpro.pdf
81 Elizabeth Outka, *Viral Modernism: The Influenza Pandemic and Interwar Literature* (Columbia University Press, 2020).
82 Emily Dickinson, *Selected Poems*, edited by Stanley Appelbaum (Dover Publications, 1990), p.5.
83 Mahmoud Darwish, 'Here the Birds' Journey Ends', *The New Yorker*, 18 August 2008, https://www.newyorker.com/magazine/2008/08/25/here-the-birds-journey-ends
84 Carlos Fuentes, *Diana: The Goddess Who Hunts Alone*, trans. Alfred Macadam (Bloomsbury Publishing, 1996), pp.39–40.
85 Suryakant Tripathi Nirala, *A Life Misspent*, trans. Satti Khanna (Harper Perennial, 2016).
86 Ibid.
87 M.K. Gandhi, *An Autobiography or the Story of My Experiments with Truth*, trans. Mahadev Desai, (Penguin, 2018), p.289.
88 Ibid.
89 Ibid., p.318.
90 Gabriel García Márquez, *The Last Interview and Other Conversations* (Melville House Publishing, 2015).
91 Ibid.
92 Daniel Defoe, *A Journal of the Plague Year* (Modern Library, 2001), p.27.
93 Ibid.
94 Max Weber, *The Protestant Ethic and the Spirit of Capitalism*, trans. Talcott Parsons (Scribner, 1958), p.117.
95 Ilan Stavans, *Gabriel García Márquez: The Early Years* (Palgrave

Macmillan, 2010), p.13.

96 Saul Bellow, *Herzog* (Penguin Classics, 2003), p.54.

97 Fifteen-year-old Churchill wrote a poem in 1890 titled 'The Influenza', on what was called the "Asiatic Flu" or the "Russian Flu" in 1889–90 and which killed over one million people worldwide. After stanzas of bad rhyme, Churchill ends the poem with these lines: 'God shield our Empire from the might / Of war or famine, plague or blight / And all the power of Hell, / And keep it ever in the hands / Of those who fought 'gainst other lands, / Who fought and conquered well.' The Empire deserved to be free from hell, so that it could freely make hell of 'other lands'. Even as an adolescent, Churchill was full of the germs of Empire, even as other germs bothered him.

98 Reviewing the film, Vincent Canby ('Satyajit Ray's Moving "Distant Thunder": The Cast', *New York Times*, 2 October 1973) observed: 'its field of vision is narrow, more or less confined to the social awakening of a young village Brahmin and his pretty, naive wife.'

99 E.M. Cioran, *A Short History of Decay* (Quartet Books, 1990), p.3.

100 Ibid., p.4.

101 Defoe, *Journal of the Plague Year*, p.13.

102 Weber writes how the advent of Calvinism ushered in an attempt 'to free man from the power of irrational impulses' and subject him 'to the supremacy of a purposeful will'. Weber, *Protestant Ethic*, p.119.

103 Ibid., p.14.

104 The reported attacks on health workers, allegedly involving members of the Tablighi Jamaat, were found to be untrue, and politically motivated (see Anon., 'Fake WhatsApp Videos Behind Attack on Health Workers in Indore: Report', *The Wire*, 3 April 2020, https://thewire.in/media/coronavirus-indore-doctors-attacked). But there were reports not involving the Jamaat, on attacks against health workers by locals in other parts of the country (Prathima Nandakumar, 'Bengaluru: Locals attack ASHA workers on COVID-19 screening duty', *The Week*, 2 April 2020, https://www.theweek.in/news/india/2020/04/02/bengaluru-locals-attack-asha-workers-covid-19-duty.html).

105 M.K. Gandhi (ed.), *Young India* (8 October 1919), https://www.gandhiheritageportal.org/journals-by-gandhiji/young-india

106 The Editors of Encyclopaedia Britannica, 'Chernobyl disaster', *Britannica*, https://www.britannica.com/event/Chernobyl-disaster; Erin Blakemore, 'The Chernobyl disaster: What happened, and the long-term impacts', *National Geographic*, 17 May 2019, https://www.nationalgeographic.com/culture/topics/reference/chernobyl-disaster/

107 Svetlana Alexievich, *Chernobyl Prayer: Voices from Chernobyl*, trans. Anna Gunin and Arc Tait (Penguin Modern Classics, 2016), p.276.

108 Ibid.

109 Ibid., p.280.

110 Octavio Paz, 'Dostoevsky: The Devil and the Ideologue,' in *On Poets and Others* (Arcade Publishing, 1990), p.101.

111 Jayanta Mahapatra, *The Whiteness of Bone* (Penguin Viking, 1992), p.43.

112 Ibid., p.44.

113 Ibid., p.46.

114 Ibid., p.45.

115 Fyodor Dostoevsky, *Demons*, trans. Robert A. Maguire (Penguin Classics, 2008), p.283.

116 Ibid., p.278.

117 Hannah Arendt, 'Thinking and Moral Considerations', in *Responsibility and Judgement* (Schocken Books, 2005), p.180.

118 John Stuart Mill, *Utilitarianism and On Liberty*, edited by M. Warnock (Fontana, 1962), p.165.

119 It included prohibitions on lust, slander and pride; encouraged virtues such as piety, prudence and kindness, and as a mark of ritual, to recite the 1,000 names of the sun in Sanskrit. The Editors of Encyclopaedia Britannica, '*Dīn-i Ilāhī*,' *Britannica*, https://www.britannica.com/topic/Din-i-Ilahi

120 In a 1901 article, Tagore engaged with what French thinker Ernest Renan wrote in his famous 1882 lecture, 'What is a Nation?', delivered at the University of Sorbonne. Tagore considered Renan's emphasis on the nation as being founded upon the shared memory of a glorious past. But, he felt a common race, or tribe, or ethnic identity (*jāti*, in India) that one finds in Europe provides a firmer foundation for the nation. India's racial or ethnic heterogeneity is a hindrance to political unity. Tagore thought India's only chance was to rely on a vague Hindu ideal of social harmony.

Tagore moved away from his own considerations of Renan's views dramatically by 1917. See Partha Chatterjee, *Lineages of Political Society* (Permanent Black, 2011), pp.94–8.

121 Tagore, 'Nationalism in the West,' p.38.

121 Ibid, p.39.

122 Ibid, p.37.

124 Mandelstam, 'The Stalin Epigram'.

125 Andrew Robinson, *Satyajit Ray: The Inner Eye* (University of California Press, 1989), p.25.

126 C.P. Cavafy, *Collected Poems*, trans. Edmund Keeley and Philip Sherrard (Chatto & Windus, 1998), p.142.

127 Ibid.

128 K. Satchidanandan, *While I Write* (HarperCollins, 2011), p.71.

129 Ibid.

130 Ibid., p.72.

131 Osip Mandelstam, *Complete Poetry of Osip Emilevich Mandelstam*, trans. Burton Raffel and Alla Burago (State University of New York Press, 1973), p.219.

132 Shakespeare's Sonnet No.138 can be traced to Montaigne. The sonnet goes:

> When my love swears that she is made of truth,
> I do believe her, though I know she lies,
> That she might think me some untutored youth,
> Unlearnèd in the world's false subtleties.
> Thus vainly thinking that she thinks me young,
> Although she knows my days are past the best,
> Simply I credit her false-speaking tongue:
> On both sides thus is simple truth suppressed.
> But wherefore says she not she is unjust?
> And wherefore say not I that I am old?
> Oh, love's best habit is in seeming trust,
> And age in love loves not to have years told.
> Therefore I lie with her and she with me,
> And in our faults by lies we flattered be.

In his essay, 'On Some Verses in Virgil', Montaigne writes, 'Lying holds an honorable place in love; it is a detour that leads us to truth by the back door.' The lovers in the sonnet follow Montaigne's assurance about 'love's best habit', where the heart reaps bountiful love, expending mere luxuries of lies. Edward A. Snow, 'Loves of Comfort and Despair: A Reading of Shakespeare's Sonnet 138,' *English Literary History*, 47:3 (Autumn 1980). I am thankful to Prasanta Chakravarty, Professor of English Literature, for bringing the Shakespeare sonnet to my notice.

133   Drew Bratcher, 'Sheltering in Place with Montaigne', *The Paris Review*, 7 April 2020, https://www.theparisreview.org/blog/2020/04/07/sheltering-in-place-with-montaigne/

134   Montaigne, *Complete Essays*, p.848.

135   Ibid., p.229.

136   'The Great Empty', *New York Times*, 23 March 2020, https://www.nytimes.com/interactive/2020/03/23/world/coronavirus-great-empty.html

137   Susan Sontag, *On Photography* (Penguin, 2002), p.16.

138   Pessoa, *Book of Disquiet*, p.148.

139   Franz Kafka, *The Diaries of Franz Kafka: 1910-1913, Volume 1*, edited by Max Brod, trans. Joseph Kresh (Schocken Books, 1948).

140   André Gide, *Journals (Volume 2: 1914-1927)*, trans. Justin O'Brien (University of Illinois Press, 2000), p.147.

141   Kafka, *Diaries of Franz Kafka*.

142   Milan Kundera, *Slowness*, trans. Linda Asher (HarperCollins, 1996), p.39.

143   Stephen Addiss, *The Art of Haiku: Its History Through Poems and Paintings by Japanese Masters* (Shambhala Publications, 2012), p.214.

144   A historian friend, Toy, told me that the gradual disappearance of Baudelaire's *flâneur* was usurped by the modern wanderer, exemplified by Jack Kerouac. The distinction, he added, is that for the *flâneur*, people (or the crowd) are the focus of attention, whereas for the wanderer, the road matters.

145   On 20 April 2020, the woman doodled something titled, 'Dreams and Reality,' which I got to see only on 23 June. I was struck by the things she described: 'heavy dreams' she can't remember when she woke up, watching trees and birds, famine that she called 'real hunger', and the

terrible situation of being caught between 'a tiny virus' and a tyrant. I was writing on some of these themes at the time. The world is more deeply connected than it thinks. Or is it that in times of crisis, human concerns converge?

146 Roland Barthes, *A Lover's Discourse: Fragments*, trans. Richard Howard (Hill and Wang, 1978), p.37.

147 Scroll Staff, 'Covid-19 lockdown: Woman rides 1,400 km on scooty to bring stranded son from Andhra Pradesh', *Scroll*, 10 April 2020, https://scroll.in/latest/958781/covid-19-lockdown-woman-rides-1400-km-on-scooty-to-bring-stranded-son-from-andhra-pradesh

148 Octavio Paz, *The Labyrinth of Solitude* (Penguin, 1985), p.197.

149 Ibid., p.198.

150 William Shakespeare, *Othello*, edited by E.A.J. Honigmann (Thomson Learning, 1997), pp.145–46.

151 Ibid., pp.146–47.

152 Ibid., p.54.

153 Sara Joe Wolansky, 'A Capital Under Quarantine in "Rome, Closed City"', *The New Yorker*, 20 March 2020, https://www.newyorker.com/culture/video-dept/a-capital-under-quarantine-in-rome-closed-city

154 Ramanujan, *Collected Poems*, p.41.

155 Aishwarya S. Iyer, '"Not Anyone's Enemy": Suicide Note of Man Targeted Over COVID-19', *The Quint*, 13 April 2020, https://www.thequint.com/news/india/mohammad-dilshad-suicide-himachal-pradesh-una-covid-19-suspicion

156 Babasaheb Ambedkar, 'Annihilation of Caste: With a Reply to Mahatma Gandhi,' in *Writings and Speeches, Volume 1* (Government of Maharashtra, 1979), p.75.

157 Ibid.

158 Yannis Ritsos, *Diaries of Exile* (Archipelago Books, 2013), p.15.

159 Ibid., p.17.

160 Ibid., p.25.

161 The oneiric aspect (and theory) of cinema has been explored by many writers and thinkers, including Roland Barthes, André Breton and Gilles Deleuze. Henri Bergson and Deleuze saw the potential for radical newness in the virtual sphere (of time and image), as the virtual exceeds

the actual by bringing past (memory) and present together in such a way that a future can be produced. Fascism has disrupted this potential, however, by distorting and policing the virtual world. Only the spectacle of lies and propaganda is being allowed to thrive.

162 Vasily Rozanov, *The Apocalypse of Our Time and other writings*, trans. Robert Pyne and Nikita Romanoff (Praeger Publishers, 1977), p.64.

163 Rimbaud, *Collected Poems*, p.253.

164 Maria Varenikova, 'Chernobyl Wildfires Reignite, Stirring Up Radiation', *New York Times*, 11 April 2020, https://www.nytimes.com/2020/04/11/world/europe/chernobyl-wildfire.html

165 Marina Tsvetaeva, *Selected Poems*, trans. Elaine Feinstein (Oxford University Press, 1971), p.46.

166 Michel Foucault et al, 'Technologies of the Self', in *Technologies of the Self: A Seminar with Michel Foucault* (University of Massachusetts Press, 1988), pp.16–49. Reproduced at https://foucault.info/documents/foucault.technologiesOfSelf.en/

167 Anon., 'PM Modi fears' (see n.27).

168 Name altered in the news report.

169 Indulekha Aravind, 'Covid-19: How healthcare workers are paying a heavy price in this battle', *The Economic Times*, 12 April 2020, https://economictimes.indiatimes.com/news/politics-and-nation/covid-19-how-healthcare-workers-are-paying-a-heavy-price-in-this-battle/articleshow/75099895.cms

170 Jeya Rani, 'An Invisible Virus Highlights the Virulence of an Age-Old Visible Virus,' *The Wire*, 14 April 2020, https://thewire.in/caste/coronavirus-caste-discrimination-india

Index

Abir 11, 168
Agyeya (Vatsyayan, Sachchidananda Hirananda) 126, 143
Akhmatova, Anna 55, 66
Alexievich, Svetlana 112
Ali, Agha Shahid 55
Ambedkar, B.R. (Babasaheb) 157
Annihilation of Caste 157
Arendt, Hannah 117
Asaf-ud-Daula 63
Assam 36, 88, 100, 133, 134, 156, 162, 175
Athens 56, 135
Aurelius, Marcus 171
Autobiography or the Story of My Experiments with Truth, An 94

Babri Masjid 16, 17
Barthes, Roland 145
Bashir, Saiyna 137
Batra, Ritesh 137
Baudelaire, Charles 6, 7, 55
Begum, Razia 146, 149
Bellow, Saul 100
Bergman, Ingmar 78
Beyond Good and Evil 79
Bezboruah, D.N. 38
Bharadwaj, Vishal 65
Bhopal 110, 114, 115
Bombay 94
Book of Disquiet, The 42, 138

Book of Laughter and Forgetting, The 28, 37, 38
Boyd, William 42
Bratcher, Drew 134, 135
Buson, Yosa 143

Caeiro, Alberto 43
Calcutta 15
Calvin, John 96
Campos, Fernando 46
Camus, Albert 7, 44
Cavafy, Constantine P. 130, 131
Chaucer, Geoffrey 86
Chernobyl 110–114, 167, 168
Chernobyl Prayer 112
Cheung, Philip 136
Chopin, Frédéric 120
Churchill, Winston 102
Cicero, Marcus Tullius 82
Cioran, E.M. 105
Coll, Maria Contreras 136
Confessions of a Mask 78

Darjeeling 76, 88, 162
Darwish, Mahmoud 56, 88
Darwish, Najwan 55
de Campos, Álvaro 46
Defoe, Daniel 95, 96, 106
Delhi 3, 13, 15, 18–23, 36, 39, 41, 42, 50, 51, 55, 62–64, 67, 68, 74–76, 87, 90, 97, 133, 137, 141, 145, 157,

159, 175
Delhi chief minister. *See:* Kejriwal, Arvind
Demeny, Paul 67
Demons. See: Devils
de Montaigne, Michel 82, 134, 135
Descartes, René 135
Devils 116
Diaries of Exile 65, 158
Dickinson, Emily 87
Dilshad Mohammad 158
Dostoevsky, Fyodor 114, 116, 117

Eisenstein, Sergei 90, 91
Eliot, T.S. 4, 9, 85–87
Engels, Fredrich 82
Esquivel, Laura 90

Faiz, Faiz Ahmed 8
Foucault, Michel 171
Fuentes, Carlos 92

Gandhi, M.K. 9, 10, 52, 94, 109, 122, 172
Gardener's Village, The. *See:* Maligaon 36
Ghosh, Sanjoy 38
Ghummakar Shastra (Treatise for the Wanderer) 144
Gide, André 140
Gitanjali 28
Godard, Jean-Luc 20, 91
Gospel According to Jesus Christ, The 43
Grass, Günter 22

Great Britain 54, 96
Guwahati 36, 37

Haavikko, Paavo 36
Hass, Robert 144
Hemingway, Ernest 25
Herbert, Zbigniew 64, 65
Herzog 100
Herzog, Werner 111
Hind Swaraj 9

Immortality 19, 28, 37
Iran 10, 45, 160

Jawaharlal Nehru University (JNU) 16, 17, 21–24, 34, 44, 76, 83, 89–92, 121–124, 141, 162, 166, 168
Jose, Lisa 175
Journal of the Plague Year, A 95, 106
Justinian 77

Kafka, Franz 50, 139, 140
Kamakhya Temple 56, 168
Kaminsky, Ilya 55
Kashmir 55, 65
Kejriwal, Arvind (Delhi chief minister) 13, 42, 63, 64
Khusro, Amir 122
Kiarostami, Abbas 5, 10, 149, 150, 160
Kolkata 15, 30, 166, 173
Kumar, Bhole 48, 49
Kumar, Jitendra 76, 80
Kumar, Kishore 23, 129
Kundera, Milan 19, 28, 37, 38, 143
Kurosawa, Akira 35

Labyrinth of Solitude, The 147
Laishram, Bidhan 34, 87, 89, 97, 162, 163
Lewis, Maria 163–167
Life is Elsewhere 38
Life Misspent, A 93
Like Water for Chocolates 90
Living to Tell the Tale 31, 82
Logesh, Balasubramani 103
Lohia, Ram Manohar 80
Loke, Atul 137
London 16, 54, 95, 106, 107, 136, 169
Love in the Time of Cholera 17
Lover's Discourse: Fragments, A 145

Mahabharata 72
Mahapatra, Jayanta 61, 62, 114–116
Maligaon 36, 163
Mallipeddi, Ramesh 21, 22, 141
Mandelstam, Osip 34, 127, 128, 133
Márquez, Gabriel García 17, 18, 20, 31, 82, 95, 96
Marx, Karl 70, 82
Melville, Jean-Pierre 20
Mill, John Stuart 117
Milosz, Czeslaw 65
Mishima, Yuko 78, 79
Modi, Narendra (Prime Minister) 13, 14, 29, 48, 64, 93, 94, 96, 97, 110, 154, 171, 174, 175
Mohammad, Dilshad 157
Monterroso, Augusto 24
Moriyama, Victor 137
Mr Lewis. *See:* Lewis, Maria
Mrs. Dalloway 54
Mumbai 6, 94, 175. *See also:* Bombay

Naipaul, V.S. 16
Nehru, Jawaharlal 34, 122, 172
Neruda, Pablo 56
New York 17–19, 46, 100, 136, 137, 167
Nietzsche, Friedrich 79, 100, 135
Nirala. *See:* Tripathi, Suryakant 54, 87, 93
Nisar, Ram Bhajan 62
Notes from Underground 116

Ojha, Krittibas 174
Old Fort. *See:* Purana Qila 55
On Liberty 117
On Photography 137
Othello 147, 148
Outka, Elizabeth 87

Padgaonkar, Dilip 15, 16
Panahi, Jafar 160, 161
Pandya, Himanshu 80, 81
Pascal, Blaise 135
Paz, Octavio 55, 69, 70, 114, 147
Peer, Basharat 65
Pessoa, Fernando 42, 43, 46, 138, 139
Plague, The 7, 44
PM (Prime Minister). *See:* Modi, Narendra
Proust, Marcel 52
Purana Qila 52, 55, 56, 60

Ramanujan, A.K. 28, 153
Ramayana 53, 72, 174
Rani, Jeya 178
Ray, Satyajit 87, 99–102, 128

Remembrance of Things Past 52
Richa 11, 14, 15, 20, 23, 25, 32, 36, 39, 46, 49, 55, 71, 97, 102, 150, 155, 156, 168
Rilke, Rainer Maria 163
Rimbaud, Arthur 67, 167
Ritsos, Yannis 56, 65, 158, 159, 160
Rome 152, 154
Rousseau, Jean-Jacques 135, 138, 172
Rozanov, Vladimir 165

Sabriée, Gilles 136
Sahu, Priyanka 60
Saint Augustine 171
Sandhu, Amandeep 33, 79, 80
Sankrityayan, Rahul 144
Saramago, José 43
Satchidanandan, K. 131
Scarpelli, Mo 152
Sebald, W.G. 41
Seberg, Jean 91, 92
Shakespeare, William 135, 147
Shantiniketan 28
Shikoh, Dara 122
Short History of Decay, A 105
Shukla, Vinod Kumar 5, 44
Simons, Marlise 18
Singh, Mohinder 76, 80, 89, 126, 127, 141, 142
Sirr-e-Akbari 122
Slowness 143

Soares, Bernardo 139, 140
Sontag, Susan 78, 102, 137
Stalin, Josef 66, 111, 127
Swaroop, Nirmal 143, 144

Tagore, Rabindranath 28, 33, 101, 123
Tarkovsky, Andrei 113
Tehran 5, 160
Testa, Andrew 136
Thoreau, David 19
Tripathi, Suryakant 'Nirala' 54
Tsvetaeva, Marina 169, 170

Unbearable Lightness of Being, The 38
United States of America 17–19, 41, 92, 95

Vatsyayan, Sachchidananda Hirananda 126
Viral Modernism: The Influenza Pandemic and Interwar Literature 87
Vyasa 72

Walden; or, Life in the Woods 19
Weber, Max 70, 96
Whiteness of Bone, The 114
Whitman, Walt 61
Woolf, Virginia 54, 55, 87, 135

Yezhov, Nicholai 66

About the author

MANASH FIRAQ BHATTACHARJEE is a poet, writer, and political science scholar from Jawaharlal Nehru University, New Delhi. He is the author of *Looking for the Nation: Towards Another Idea of India* (Speaking Tiger, 2018) and a collection of poetry, *Ghalib's Tomb and Other Poems* (The London Magazine, 2013). He frequently writes for the *Wire*, and has contributed to the *New York Times*, *Al-Jazeera*, *Los Angeles Review of Books*, *Guernica*, the *Hindu*, the *Indian Express*, *Outlook*, among other publications. His poetry has appeared in *Rattle*, *World Literature Today*, *Acumen*, the *Fortnightly Review*, among others. He has taught lyric poetry and literary journalism at Ambedkar University, New Delhi.